THE RUNNER'S GUIDE TO
HEALTHY
FEET AND
ANKLES

THE RUNNER'S GUIDE TO
HEALTHY
FEET AND
ANKLES

SIMPLE STEPS TO PREVENT INJURY AND RUN STRONGER

BRIAN W. FULLEM, DPM

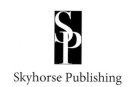

Skyhorse Publishing

Skyhorse Publishing books may be purchased in bulk at special discounts for sales promotion, corporate gifts, fund-raising, or educational purposes. Special editions can also be created to specifications. For details, contact the Special Sales Department, Skyhorse Publishing, 307 West 36th Street, 11th Floor, New York, NY 10018 or info@ skyhorsepublishing.com.

Skyhorse® and Skyhorse Publishing® are registered trademarks of Skyhorse Publishing, Inc.®, a Delaware corporation.

Visit our website at www.skyhorsepublishing.com.

10 9 8 7 6 5 4 3 2 1

Library of Congress Cataloging-in-Publication Data is available on file.

Cover design by Tom Lau
Cover photo credit: iStockphoto

Photos by Brian W. Fullem, unless otherwise noted.

Print ISBN: 978-1-5107-0894-5
Ebook ISBN: 978-1-5107-0896-9

Printed in China

Contents

Foreword

How to stay healthy? Or, if you're a pessimist, how not to get injured?

That's the quandary most runners face, and largely what the running industry is about.

Running shoes, running technique, stretching techniques, icing techniques, how to warm up, how to cool down, foam rollers, compression gear . . . the list goes on and on of things that are supposed to keep us runners healthy and on the roads and trails.

I've been a runner for the majority of my life. I've progressed from trying to run the entirety of PE class in first grade for some unknown reason, to spending four years of my life trying to make the Olympics, to just enjoying running with my dogs along the river. You'd think that after all these years of running and being a self-proclaimed "expert" at LetsRun.com, that I'd know how to stay healthy, but I don't have a clue.

One thing I do know: the human body may have been perfectly designed to run long distances, but it wasn't perfectly designed to run mile after mile in a straight line, especially on pavement.

That is why I got excited when I heard Brian Fullem was writing *The Runner's Guide to Healthy Feet and Ankles*. Brian is not only a lifelong runner, but also a top-notch podiatrist. It's a rare combination: a person who understands everything about runners and what we're trying to do, and understands the body and how our feet, ankles, and everything else works. There isn't a better person to write *The Runner's Guide to Healthy Feet and Ankles* than him.

I first met Brian online. At the time, I was confounded by pain in my heel and was at a loss as to what to do. Having tried various remedies and seen a few people, I did what anyone else who has started an online running community does—I posted about my frustrations there.

Brian replied with some advice I had not seen elsewhere and suggested I see him when I happened to be in Boston. I saw him and received immediate relief for my condition. That started our professional relationship, which also turned into a friendship. I soon started recommending other people see Brian as well, and soon my brother, who was the distance coach at Cornell University at the time, was driving four hours with some of his athletes to see Brian.

Brian doesn't have miracle cures for everyone, and isn't afraid to admit when he doesn't. But he always has a sound course of action and a commitment to figuring out the problem. Brian doesn't push surgery, but isn't afraid of it, and willing to recommend when someone needs it. I think that's a great combination because Brian's first inclination is to get you healthy rather than put you under the knife. Even better than dealing with injuries is preventing them, and that's the main reason I recommend *The Runner's Guide to Healthy Feet and Ankles* to every runner.

—Weldon Johnson, co-founder of LetsRun.com
and former Olympic hopeful at 10,000 meters

Introduction

The Importance of Healthy Feet and Ankles for Runners

Running is a lifestyle choice for millions of people, and one of the best and easiest ways to exercise. Unfortunately, more than half of all runners will experience an injury at some point in their running career. Some injuries are simple matters that resolve quickly, while others are more complex and might not resolve just by taking a few days off from running.

This book will provide a road map to help you navigate the most common running injuries, along with tips on prevention, home remedies, and advice as to when it's appropriate to seek treatment from a medical specialist. Much of the advice in this book is based on high-level medical evidence that has been published in peer-reviewed journals, along with my twenty-plus years as a sport podiatrist and my own experience as a competitive runner (which, full disclosure, has included many of the injuries in this book).

Some doctors tell runners they should stop training completely with just about every injury. That's not my approach.

In my practice and in this book, my goal is to help runners keep running. Of course, there are times when taking a break from running is unavoidable, but that should never be the only treatment. The focus of sports medicine should always be to help prevent injury, to find and treat the cause of the injury if a runner is hurt and not just treat the symptoms. In this book, I'll show you how to treat an injury at home initially, give guidance on when to see a sports medicine specialist, and tell you how to keep the problem from recurring.

Feet First

It's obvious that your feet and ankles play a huge role in your running. So at the outset, let's take a general look at these important body parts, and what exactly they do when you run.

The foot is a complex structure with twenty-eight bones, thirty-three joints, and many muscles and tendons, a majority of which originate in the lower leg. An excellent analogy is that the feet are vital to the body in a similar manner as that of the basement to the house—if the basement isn't providing a proper foundation, then the house may fall apart.

There are three distinct phases of the running gait cycle when the foot is on the ground: foot strike, mid-stance, and toe-off. There has been some debate in the running community about which part of the foot should strike first, with a recent movement to get people away from heel striking. However, there's no proof that landing on the heel hinders performance, and no correlation has been shown between heel striking and increased injury risk.

More important is where your foot lands in relation to your body's center of gravity. Ideally, your foot lands as close to directly under your body as possible. Landing far in front of your center of gravity, or overstriding, might increase the impact forces of running, which may increase your susceptibility to injury.

I don't advise runners to change their method of foot strike without a good reason, as I have found that simple changes can sometimes lead to injury. For example, a recent trend was to transition runners away from heel striking to spend more time on the forefoot, which has the side effect of stressing the Achilles and leading to an increase in Achilles tendon injuries. If you're experiencing repeated injuries that may be associated with landing with too much impact, then that might warrant a slight change in your foot strike pattern. A good course of action would be to attempt to land "softer" to lessen the impact. You can practice landing with less impact by finding a nice grass field and performing some strides barefoot; without the protection of shoes, your body will adjust its landing to be less on the heel to lessen the impact forces.

Following heel strike is midstance, when the foot is fully on the ground. The final phase is toe-off, or propulsion.

After the foot strikes the ground, a series of actions occur in sequence; if any portion of that sequence is out of alignment, then it will impact the next phase. Most runners will be familiar with the terms "pronation" and "supination." Old medical dogma identified overpronation as a cause of running injuries. It's currently proposed in much of the new medical literature that there's no such thing as overpronation—the theory is that the foot pronates as much as the body needs and what the motions of the foot will allow.

Simply put, pronation occurs when the foot is rolling in towards the midline of the body. It is a motion that occurs in three planes or directions. The body requires a certain amount of pronation in the foot to help absorb shock at impact. The technical aspect of what occurs in foot pronation is eversion

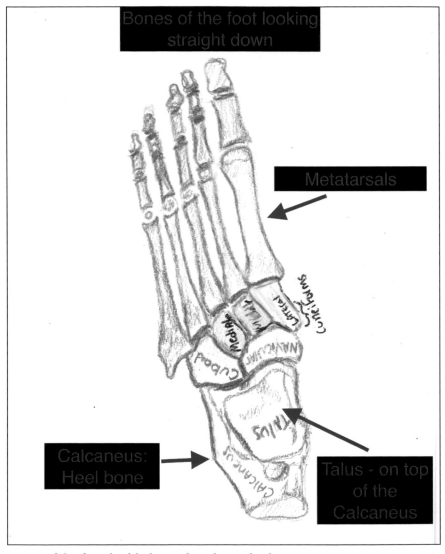

Bones of the foot, highlighting the talus and calcaneus.

Drawing by Annemarie Fullem, PT

of the calcaneus, where the heel bone tilts in towards the midline of the body, along with adduction and plantarflexion of the talus, the bone on top of the calcaneus.

Supination is the opposite motion, and occurs before propulsion. During supination the foot rolls to the outside as the calcaneus inverts and the talus abducts and dorsiflexes. Supination and pronation have an effect on the rest of the body, particularly when the foot is in contact with the ground; this is known as closed chain kinetics or biomechanics.

When the foot is pronating while on the ground, the leg will internally rotate, placing stress on the knee, hips, and back. If the foot does not pronate enough to absorb shock, then that force must be attenuated higher up the leg and may lead to pain in the structures above the foot, such as shin or knee pain. This can occur if a runner is in a shoe that controls too much motion or if an insert is in the shoe that stops too much pronation. Pronation unlocks the foot to allow the absorption of impact forces, while supination serves to lock the foot in order to form a rigid lever to help provide a stable structure to push off properly.

Each time your foot strikes the ground during a run, it will have an impact of two to four times your body weight. Many running injuries are overuse-type injuries, but there are many factors that can lead to an injury, including running shoes, choice of running surface, whether your foot strikes the ground with the heel, midfoot, or forefoot, and other factors that we will explore in depth later in this book.

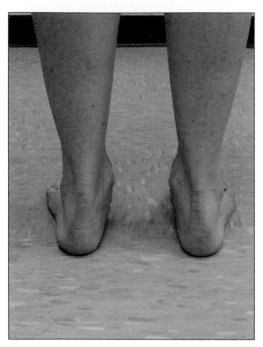

The feet from behind showing a more pronated position.

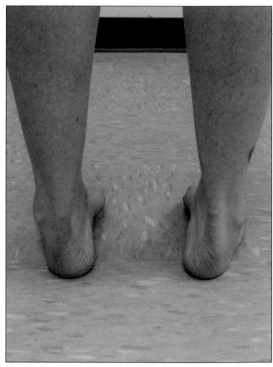

The feet in a supinated position.

Advice About Advice

Throughout this book, I'll be providing guidance on how to proceed if you have one of the many injuries runners can get. But first, here's some advice that applies to any injured runner, regardless of the location or type of injury.

A good general rule is that if you're limping, then you shouldn't be running. Some may not think or even realize they are limping, but if you're experiencing consistent pain while running, then chances are that your body will begin to compensate to alleviate the stress on the injured area, often times subconsciously. When your feet, ankles, or legs are in pain during a run for more than a couple of days, it's often best to take a few days off to see if the area improves.

If there's swelling, or the pain doesn't subside, consider seeing your local sports podiatrist. You can ask running friends for a referral; if they don't know anyone, then call your local running specialty store and see if they can make a recommendation.

The American Academy of Podiatric Sports Medicine (AAPSM) certifies podiatrists who have a special interest in sports medicine topics and treatments. The highest level of certification, known as fellowship status, is a good indicator of a podiatrist who will provide better care to athletes. Becoming a fellow of the AAPSM requires taking a written exam and providing evidence of work in the sports medicine field, including serving as a team physician for a local sports team and lecturing to the public and other physicians. The organization's website, www.AAPSM.org, provides a great deal of excellent information as well as a list of all the podiatrists who have attained fellowship status.

If possible, see a specialist like a fellow of the AAPSM who understands how to treat athletes, as some physicians think running is inadvisable when injured, and their advice will be to stop running. A good physician listens to and works in conjunction with the patient to develop a treatment plan and a safe return to running after providing a proper diagnosis and treatment plan that addresses the cause of the injury and not just the symptoms.

I try to never tell my patients that they can't run or participate in their sport unless there's a valid reason, such as a stress fracture or a similar debilitating injury. As the saying goes, when life hands you lemons, make lemonade. When you're injured, try to view the time as an opportunity to shore up your weaknesses, and work on your strength and flexibility with activities that don't cause pain. We will discuss the proper strengthening, stretching, alternative exercises, and tools that can be used to stay healthy, prevent future injuries, and recover from your current injuries in this book.

About the Author

I'd like to end this introduction by, well, introducing myself. I hope that, by reading about my running and professional background, you'll better understand where I'm coming from in the advice you'll find throughout this book.

I began running at a young age, attempting to follow in my older brother's footsteps. I loved all sports, but whether it was basketball, baseball, or any other sport, the running aspect was my best attribute. I ran my first races before I was ten years old, and my love for the sport grew as I was lucky enough to grow up during the running boom fostered by Frank Shorter's win in the 1972 Olympic Marathon.

Growing up in Utica, New York also provided a boost, as the running community was very supportive and strong even before I ran the first Utica Boilermaker 15K Road race in 1978. (The race now attracts more than 14,000 runners every July.) I had great coaching at Notre Dame High School by Rich Ambruso and finished fifth in the 3,200 meters at the NYS Track Championships in 9:19 as a junior and third in the NYS Cross Country Champs as a senior in 1981. I loved every aspect of the sport and read as many training books as I could get my hands on, subscribed to *Runner's World* and *Running Times*, and read most of Dr. George Sheehan's books, which were more about the philosophical aspects of running than the actual physical act.

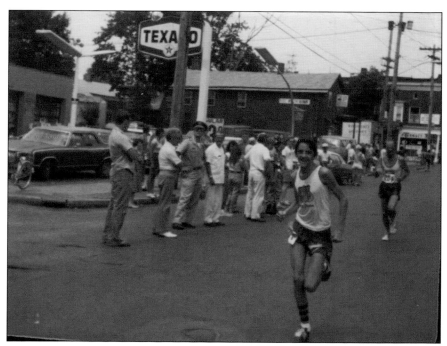

Dr. Fullem at age thirteen, running the 1978 Utica Boilermaker 15K.
Photo by Bill Fullem

I continued my running at Bucknell University under the tutelage of Coach Art Gulden. At Bucknell, I ran most of my personal bests, including 3:52 for 1,500 meters, 8:50 for 2 miles, and 14:25 for 5,000 meters. These days, degenerative changes in my left knee (unrelated to running) prevent me from running every day, but I still continue to love to run.

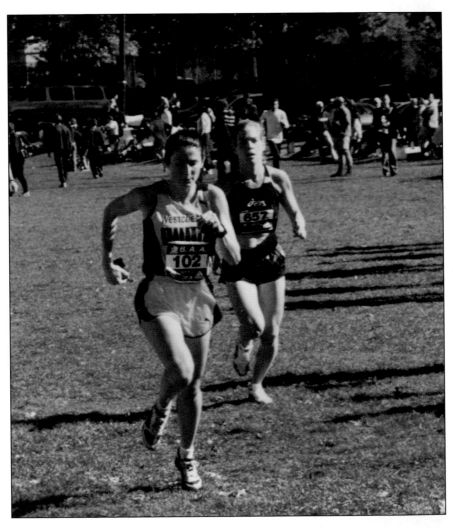

Annemarie Fullem running cross country at Franklin Park in Boston.

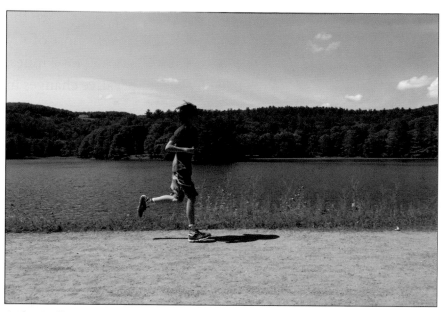

Aidan Fullem running as a thirteen-year-old.

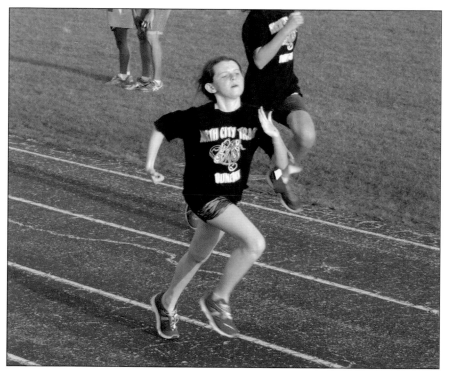

Erin Fullem running track as an eleven-year-old.

Much of the good in my life directly stems from running, including my profession and my family. While running for the Westchester Track Club in New York for Coach Mike Barnow, I met Annemarie, my wife of more than sixteen years. Annemarie is the school record holder at Hunter College in New York City in the indoor and outdoor 1,500 meters, and she finished ninth in the DIII Outdoor NCAA Championships in 1993. She is now a physical therapist and, like me, is able to combine her love of running with her profession. We have two children, Aidan and Erin, who have both competed in track and cross country. We hope they'll continue to run for the rest of their lives, if only for the health benefits.

My competitive career in running spanned more than thirty years and, combined with the treatment of athletes of all levels, has allowed me to be uniquely qualified to provide advice and treat any running injury in the lower extremities.

My journey towards becoming a sports medicine podiatrist began when I hurt my foot while running an indoor track race at Bucknell. I was diagnosed with plantar fasciitis, but in retrospect, the injury was most likely a tear of the fascia. It was the first serious injury of my running career, and it fostered my resolve to want to help athletes, and runners in particular. After twenty-five years in practice I still enjoy spending a significant portion of my time treating injured runners and helping them get back to doing what they enjoy. It's my hope that this book allows runners to stay healthy and, when injured, to get healthy.

Chapter One

Running Shoes and Orthotic Devices

The only piece of equipment that a runner really needs is a good pair of running shoes. That said, other things, such as choice of socks or inserts for the shoes, can help you stay healthier and have a better running experience.

My general advice is that once you find a brand or model of shoe that works well for you, then stick with it. Often an injury is preceded by a change in shoe brand or style. There's no best shoe for everyone, but there is a best shoe for each person. In this chapter, we'll look at how to find the right shoe for you, and what to consider about the other items underfoot when you run.

The Parts of a Running Shoe

Let's start by examining the different components of a running shoe. The "last" of a shoe refers to its shape. It's best determined by looking at the shape of the shoe from the bottom. Most running shoes are now built with a semi-curved last to mimic the shape of the foot. Some shoes, such as the Brooks Dyad, have a straighter edge along the inside, which provides more stability. I've found this type of shoe can work well for a runner with a flatter foot who doesn't do well with a traditional stability or motion-control shoe.

The back of the shoe is the heel counter. In theory, a firmer counter makes the shoe more stable, but a hard heel counter can cause irritation to the back of a runner's heel, especially if there are any boney prominences as in a Haglund's deformity.

The upper is the part of the shoe that covers the top of the foot. Shoe companies have significantly improved uppers. Many are now seamless, which has helped remove parts of the shoe that could cause blisters and painful pressure spots.

The midsole is the cushioned section below your foot. It can be made of different materials, including ethyl vinyl acetate (EVA), which tends to be softer and makes the shoe feel more cushioned but wears out faster, and polyurethane (PU), which can feel firmer and is heavier but is often more durable than EVA. There are also some newer materials that show great promise in providing cushioning while possibly improving performance. An example of this next-generation midsole material is Adidas Boost. In one high-quality medical study comparing the Adidas Boost to another brand, the Boost was found to improve oxygen consumption in athletes by a small amount. The Boost uses a different formulation of PU than that used in conventional midsoles. Adidas claims it maintains its original shape better than EVA and standard PU.

The final component of the shoe is the outsole, which is the part that makes direct contact with the ground. It's often composed of carbon rubber or a softer blown rubber. The outsole can help to provide traction, such as when a waffle-type sole is used, or can be smoother, such as in a road racing flat. Blown rubber may provide a softer ride but will also wear out faster.

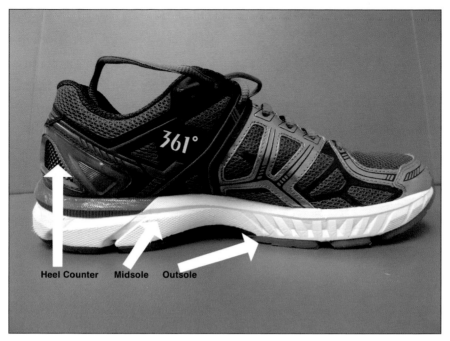

Heel Counter   Midsole   Outsole

Components of the running shoe: outsole, midsole, heel counter, and upper.

Categories of Shoes

Running shoes are often divided into three main types: neutral, stability, and motion control. These categories are useful for the purpose of a broad overview, but as we'll see below, I disagree with the idea of pigeonholing people with a given foot type into the same category of shoe.

The neutral shoe is traditionally a cushioned shoe with no motion-control properties, and softer material in the midsole of the shoe. The stability shoe provides some medial posting of the shoe with a firmer density material in the midsole on the inside of the shoe. "Posting" refers to extra material added to the midsole in an attempt to partially limit the amount of pronation, or inward motion of the foot. We'll revisit posting when looking at orthotic devices later in this chapter.

The third category is motion-control shoes, which are typically heavier and have much firmer medial midsole materials that sometimes incorporate hard plastic to significantly control pronation. I rarely recommended a motion-control shoe, and most companies have moved away from extreme motion-control properties. Still, there are some runners who do better with this type of shoe, especially bigger runners.

What's known as "the wet test" has been touted as a way to determine what type of running shoe to buy. It involves looking at the footprint you leave on something like a tiled bathroom floor when your feet are wet. If your footprint shows more of your arch than foot in contact with the ground, then you supposedly need more control from your shoe. A higher arch leaves less of a footprint, and that foot type is said to require more cushioning. A foot type somewhere in the middle of those two should be in a stability shoe, according to proponents of the wet test.

This test provides a good general guide as to discerning which shoe category might be best for your particular foot type, and can help beginning runners with a starting point of which shoes to try on initially. But the test shouldn't completely determine which type of shoe you choose. For example, as we'll see later in this chapter, a person with a flat foot might feel best in a neutral shoe.

Maximalist and minimalist are two relatively new types of shoes that deserve consideration. An example of the most minimalist shoe is the Vibram FiveFingers. The category isn't particularly well-defined, but generally includes shoes that are lighter with less midsole material. Hoka One One helped to start the maximalist shoe category with a shoe that features up to twice the normal midsole cushioning material than a traditional running shoe. I view all the new shoes as a welcome addition providing more choices for runners to find the best model for them.

With the popularity of the book *Born to Run* by Christopher McDougall in 2009, a lot of runners have switched to minimalist shoes. For many, the ultimate goal was to run barefoot; sales of FiveFingers soared because the shoe closely mimics being unshod.

Some people failed to realize that adjusting to a minimalist or barefoot shoe requires a change in foot strike. There wasn't an increase in injuries for people who switched to those types of shoes, but there was a significant spike of different types of injuries. I believe that this was due to an attempt at changing foot-strike patterns too soon without a transition period, and to the fact that not every runner is going to be able to adapt to this approach. In my practice I saw an increase in sesamoid and forefoot injuries as well fractures of bones such as the cuboid, which is usually broken only by a traumatic injury.

Some of my injured patients will also attempt to switch their running form and go to a more minimalist shoe on the advice of others that it will improve their performance. Keep in mind that the medical literature doesn't show any evidence that changing from being a heel striker to more of a forefoot striker will have any impact on improving performance. A study of the foot-strike patterns of the top ten finishers at the 2011 Boston Marathon found that some landed on the heel, some on the front of the foot, and others landed midfoot. I am not completely against barefoot or minimalist-type shoes. But—and I can't emphasize this strongly enough—if you're healthy and not having injury problems, there's really no need to change your type of shoes or foot-strike pattern.

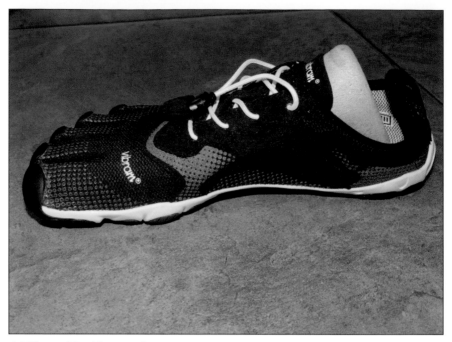

A Vibram FiveFingers shoe.

While I typically don't recommend barefoot or minimalist running to my patients, I think some may benefit from it, especially if traditional running shoes are leading to injury problems. One sports medicine expert who does recommend minimalist shoes for his patients is Dr. Mark Cucuzzella. He's a family practice medical doctor with an emphasis on helping his patients to exercise pain-free. Dr. Cucuzzella found that when his patients had injury problems that they could not overcome in traditional running shoes, they were able to run in minimalist shoes or barefoot with great success when given good instruction on how to transition to and run in less shoe. Dr. Cucuzzella's opinion is strengthened by his personal experience—he says he runs pain-free barefoot or in minimalist shoes, and he ran under 3:00 in the marathon in his late forties.

The red-hot days of the barefoot and minimalist craze are over. One positive to come from it: more mainstream shoes have incorporated minimalism's emphasis on less of a difference between the height of the heel and the height of the forefoot.

This measurement is sometimes called the heel drop or ramp angle of the shoe. Most running shoe companies had set

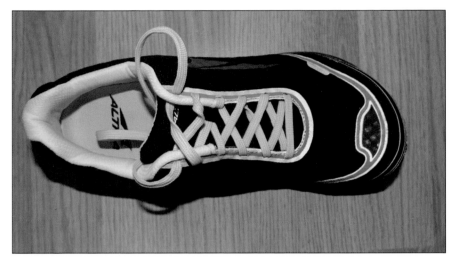

An Altra running shoe.

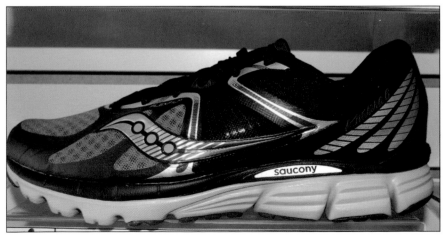

A Saucony running shoe.

their training shoes at a 12 mm differential, which can lead to more stress on the forefoot structures as well as other adaptive issues that alters one's mechanics. Many of the companies are now adding other options with a lower heel height. Saucony has lowered their highest differential from 12 mm to 8 mm. Some companies like Altra tout a zero differential in the majority of their shoes. Some experts feel that a shoe with no differential or zero drop allows a runner to run more efficiently, but be careful about switching immediately from a 12 mm shoe to a zero drop. The change should take place gradually; a good running specialty store should be able to help you find choices between the two extremes.

As mentioned above, Hoka One One has helped to create a whole new category of running shoes, the maximalist shoe. Hoka added more cushioning along with a rocker-type curve on the bottom of the shoe, which can be an excellent choice

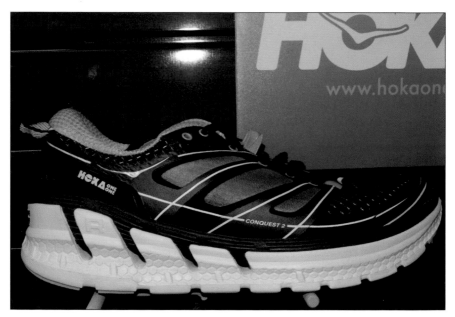

A Hoka One One running shoe.

for those who need less pressure in the front of the foot or feel best with extra cushioning. Several shoe companies are now offering this option of models with more of what's known as stack height, or how much midsole material sits between your foot and the ground. Patients with forefoot pain such as hallux limitus can benefit from this style of shoe. Hokas and other maximalist models don't give the feeling that you're elevated or unstable. Part of that comes from the fact that even these thickly cushioned shoes have a fairly small heel-to-toe drop.

Altra is another unique option, as besides the zero drop they feature a wider toe box, which allows more room in the forefoot. I sometimes recommend a patient try Altras when they have issues with the width of the shoe. Examples include a neuroma being aggravated or a bunion deformity that can

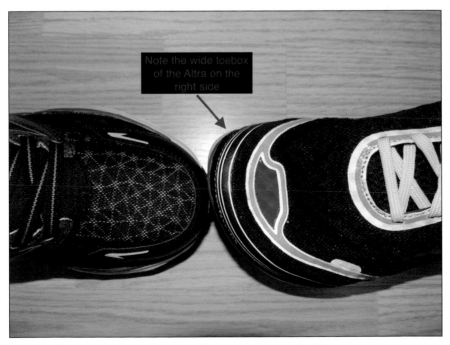

An Altra's toe box shape compared to another brand of shoe.

be aggravated in a shoe with a normal width or traditional tapered-at-the-front shape.

MBT has a line of running shoes that feature a rocker-like sole. In the past, they've offered this type of shoe as a medical option. People with arthritis in the big toe joint, known as hallux limitus or hallux rigidus, may benefit from these shoes.

Where to Buy Running Shoes

The best place to buy new shoes is a specialty running store. I always recommend supporting local running stores because they'll provide good advice and, ideally, help you find the proper shoe for your unique needs.

It is always best to try a shoe on first before purchasing. Another reason to visit the running specialty store is for the right fit, as a size 9 for one shoe company may be a size 10 in another. Even among models within the same company there can be great variability.

If possible, do a little running around the parking lot or on a store's treadmill before purchasing. The better stores will even encourage a test run. Some of the bigger box stores will try to sell you an extra arch support or other potentially unnecessary products when you buy a new pair of shoes. If you're not having any injury issues, there's no need for an extra arch support.

Keep in mind that smaller stores will have a lower inventory of shoes and choices across models. For example, some models come in three or four widths, but not all will be available. Online options provide a wider range of choices, and if you already know that a particular make and model fits you well, then purchasing online might be a good option. Be wary of buying the next year's version of the same model without the opportunity to try it on. Sometimes there are enough changes to make the newer model fit and feel very differently.

Finding the Right Shoe for You

Runners will sometimes choose a shoe that's too small, as it seems to be the proper fit in the store, but isn't once you're running. One good rule for choosing the proper length of a shoe: leave a space that measures the length of your thumbnail from the end of your longest toe (which can sometimes be the second toe instead of your big toe) to the end of the shoe.

The shoe should be perfectly comfortable initially with no uncomfortable spots. Make sure the heel counter feels comfortable and isn't too firm against the back of your heel. Also make sure the shoe feels wide enough to accommodate to the widest part of your foot, and, if you wear an orthotic insert, that the shoe is deep enough. Feet tend to swell a bit during the day so the ideal fitting time is probably midday, but if you run early in the morning or at the end of the day, you might want to synch your shoe testing with when you usually run.

Dr. Benno Nigg is one of the top researchers in the world regarding how running shoes interact with the feet and legs. In a study he published in 2015, Dr. Nigg wrote that there's no evidence in the medical literature from the last forty years that running shoes can prevent injury. He also noted that running shoes have little effect on altering the motion of the foot. Dr. Nigg wrote that people will move in their preferred movement pathway regardless of the motion control or lack of motion-control properties in the shoes.

The most important aspect of this paper may be that if people are more comfortable in their running shoes then they have fewer injuries. The take-home point when shoe shopping: Try on shoes and let comfort be your first priority. Don't completely follow the conventional advice based on your foot type or motion of the foot that some stores may offer. At least as important is that the shoe feels like an extension of your foot.

Keep in mind that every shoe company has a different idea of what the typical foot shape is and how the shoe should be manufactured. Some companies may have a narrower last while others may be wider. It's usually best to remain in the same company's shoes, but some companies' shoes are more compatible across brands than others. For example, I've found that Nike and Mizuno tend to fit similarly to each other, as do Brooks and Asics.

There may be some benefit to using two different shoes, either a different model of the same brand or models from two brands. One recent medical study of 264 recreational runners followed for over a year revealed that the runners who wore only one brand and type of shoe suffered 37 percent more injuries than the group that alternated shoes. Runners in the latter group wore one pair at most 58 percent of the time. The conclusion of the study was that alternating different shoe models leads to different areas being stressed, which in turn lowers your injury risk.

Socks

Socks may seem simple, but there are a lot of options. At a minimum, runners should be using a microfiber-type material such as CoolMax, which whisks the moisture away from the foot so that it can evaporate quickly. Cotton socks absorb and retain moisture, which can lead to blisters and other hygienic issues such as an athlete's foot infection. Wool produces the least friction and has the benefit of providing a warmer environment for the feet, but it absorbs more moisture than blends and microfiber socks. A wool blend in the winter is a good choice for warmth and reducing the chance of blisters. But they may retain too much moisture for use in the summer, making them feel heavier and, like wet cotton socks, potentially increasing the chance of an athlete's foot infection.

Besides the material the socks are made of, personal preference should guide other aspects of sock choice, including thickness and length. Brands such as Thorlo make socks with thicker padding in the heel or forefoot to better absorb shock. Brands such as Wright make double-layered socks designed to help reduce blisters.

There's very little medical evidence concerning the use of socks to help prevent injury. Studies from the military have not shown any indication that sock choice can reduce injuries. My advice is to wear a moisture-wicking fabric in a thickness you prefer and find comfortable.

Compression socks up to the knees have garnered a lot of interest as of late, as elite runners such as Meb Keflezighi and Shalane Flanagan are seen wearing them during competitions. The medical literature hasn't shown any evidence that the socks can improve performance, but there is proof that wearing them post-workout or post-race can help improve recovery. A recent study of Australian marathoners showed an improved performance by runners using compression socks after the marathon in a treadmill test, when compared to those in the placebo group. The conclusion of the study was that the compression sock allowed faster recovery, which

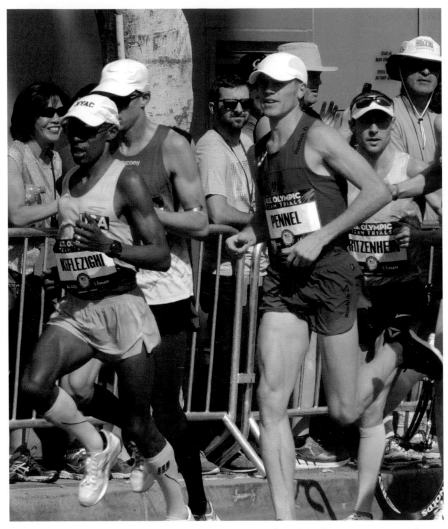

Meb Keflezighi at the 2016 U.S. Olympic Marathon Trials en route to making his fourth Olympic team.

can translate into better subsequent performance due to being able to return to normal training sooner. There's no downside to wearing compression socks, so if you feel better using them during training or racing, then by all means continue to wear them.

Inserts and Custom Orthotic Devices

As a podiatrist, I often treat runners who wonder if they'll benefit from orthotics. The simple answer is to consider the use of a foot orthotic device if you have an injury or a series of injuries that aren't improving with other treatments. I rarely recommend a custom orthotic device for a runner who doesn't have a history of injury.

A foot orthotic device is designed to help support and alter the motions of the foot in order to help heal or prevent injuries. The devices are divided into two categories, over-the-counter (OTC) and custom. Some companies advertise "custom fit," or make similar claims for their OTC devices. Beware of stores that advertise they will cure your arch and heel pain; their main goal is to separate you from your money. A true custom device involves creating an impression of the foot, after which a prescription is

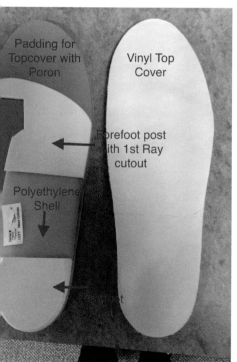

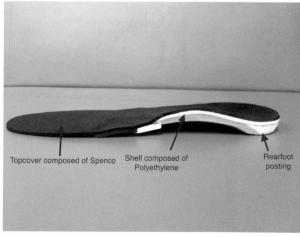

Custom orthotics, showing the various components.

developed to instruct the lab on modifications such as posting, additional padding or cutouts, as well as what materials to use for the shell or body of the device.

If you're experiencing an injury that could be related to your foot function, such as heel pain or tendonitis in the outside or inside of the ankles, then it might be worth trying an OTC device first to see how you respond before going to the doctor.

I often recommend an OTC device initially. In my office, I dispense Powerstep insoles. Other brands I've found to be reliable include SuperFeet, Spenco, and Sof Sole. An OTC device shouldn't cost more than $40 to $50 in most cases. The advantage of these devices is minimal cost, but they might not work well for someone with an unusually high or flat arch height.

If you have pain in the ball of the foot, you can add some padding to the OTC insert to help remove more pressure away from the painful area. Similarly, padding in the form of 1/8" or

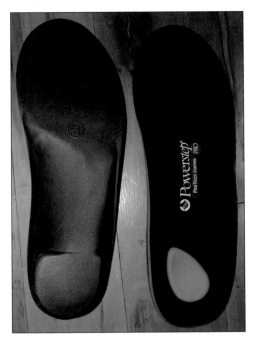

1/16" adhesive felt can be added to the bottom of the insert to tilt the foot in or out. Adhesive felt padding can be purchased online in thicknesses ranging from 1/32" (which is called Moleskin) up to 1/8". I most commonly use 1/8" adhesive felt to pad different areas and to make accommodations on inserts.

Powerstep insoles.

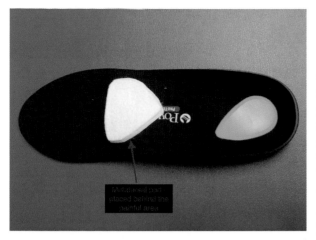

Over-the-counter insert with metatarsal padding, 1/8" adhesive felt cut into a heart-shaped pad. The pad should be behind the area where the pain is located, not directly under the painful spot.

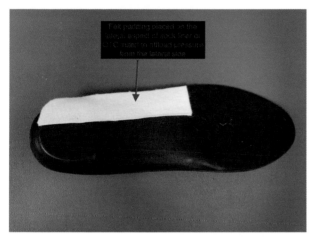

Over-the-counter insert with 1/8" felt padding along the outside edge to tilt the foot inwards to alleviate pain from the lateral side of the foot, such as in peroneal tendonitis.

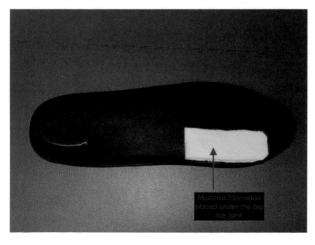

Over-the-counter insert with a 1/8" felt Morton's extension for pain in the big toe joint when it bends.

In most cases it's best to remove the insert that comes with shoes if you're using an OTC or custom orthotic device. Leaving the sock liner in will make the shoe too tight. You might need to switch to a bigger shoe size to accommodate a custom orthotic device. For this reason I always recommend trying on new shoes with whatever insert you're currently using before buying a new model or brand.

Custom foot orthotics can be a valuable treatment in some injuries, but the challenge is deciding how and when to use this sometimes over-prescribed treatment. Also keep in mind that they can be expensive and are often not covered by insurance. Another important caveat: there are times in my practice when I see an athlete who has been wearing custom devices for years and cannot recall why he or she is wearing them. Occasionally, I will advise the patient to transition out of the devices.

My philosophy on custom orthotic devices is simply that they're not a cure-all and not everyone needs to have them fabricated, but some people can definitely benefit from them. Custom devices can incorporate different modifications and multiple layers of material. In some cases, custom devices will prove more effective than an OTC device because it will match up better to your foot and arch, and modifications can be tailored to your specific foot and injury.

Your podiatrist should consider several factors in choosing the proper device to fabricate for your feet, including the location of the injury, your foot type, and your past history with inserts. Certain injuries respond very well to a custom orthotic. Arch pain, plantar fasciitis (heel pain), shin splints, and pain in the tendons along the inside (posterior tibial tendon) and outside of the ankle (peroneal tendons) are all ailments that may improve with a custom device.

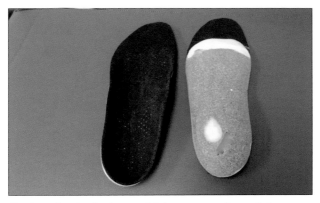

Cork orthotic devices, which support the arch better in some cases.

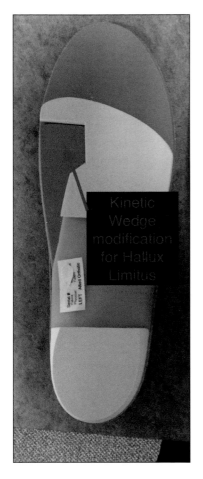

Custom orthotic with kinetic wedge cutout, a good device and modification choice for hallux limitus and big toe joint pain.

Foot type should also play a part in the decision to add a custom insert to the treatment plan. In general, a flatter foot can sometimes benefit from a more rigid device, while a higher-arched foot may respond better to a more cushioned device.

It's commonly accepted that plantar fasciitis is partly due to the insertion of the fascia pulling away from the attachment in the heel. An insert can help take some of the tension off the plantar fascia and hopefully allow it to heal.

In shin splints (medically known as medial tibial stress syndrome), the posterior tibial tendon is one of the two main muscles that is overworked and a cause of the injury. The posterior tibial tendon functions partly to invert the foot and partly to help the foot maintain arch height. An orthotic device can remove part of the load on this important tendon.

An orthotic device for peroneal tendon pain will be designed a little differently than devices for other injuries, in that it will tilt the foot more to the inside to take the pressure off the peroneal tendons.

Two injuries that I almost never recommend a custom orthotic device for are iliotibial band syndrome and medial (inner part of the leg) knee pain. Older medical literature will often recommend a custom orthotic device for these injuries, but the opposite is usually preferable. These injuries respond better when the motion of the foot is not restricted too much.

If you have a running injury but are pain-free during your non-running hours, it might be best if the custom orthotic is only worn for training. One negative aspect of the custom devices is that the intrinsic foot muscles can become weaker from being constantly supported. For this reason, athletes who wear orthotics should do strengthening exercises for the feet. Two simple exercises are to grab a towel with your toes, raise it up off the ground and hold for five seconds. Build up to two sets of holding the towel for 15 seconds at a time. A second exercise is to lay a towel flat with a five-pound weight or book at the other end and use your toes to scrunch up the towel, pulling the weighted end towards you. (More on foot strengthening in Chapter 6.)

The fabrication of a custom device is the most important aspect of the device. There are three main casting methods:

computerized scanning, foam impression, and plaster casting. In my opinion, plaster casting is the most reliable and best method. A foam impression box makes it difficult to hold the foot in the proper position, and the scanners make any abnormalities difficult to capture.

In my practice, I have the patient lay prone on my exam table. Then I use plaster to create my impression of the foot while holding the foot in a corrected position. The quality of the cast determines how well the device will work, so in most cases the casting should be performed only by the physician, not by a medical assistant. The cast is then sent to an orthotic laboratory. It often takes several weeks before the devices arrive.

The doctor should collaborate with you on the best type of materials, the posting, and length of the device. Two important aspects that should always be the goal when prescribing a custom orthotic device are that the device is comfortable and helps you become pain-free. The medical literature has shown that custom orthotic devices can alter the forces that are acting on the foot and reduce pressures to certain areas. The force acting on the foot is known as ground reaction force, which can be altered with different modifications when fabricating a custom orthotic device.

A gradual break-in process should take place over a two- to three-week period. Run in new orthotics only after they're comfortable to walk around in. Again, if you are experiencing pain only while running, then after that initial break in-period orthotic devices should need to be worn only while working out.

If the devices don't feel comfortable, they sometimes require an adjustment. Most commonly the arch height might need to be lowered or posting materials might have to be adjusted. Occasionally a different pair may need to be fabricated, such as if you can't tolerate a firmer device, even if that's what is typically used for your injury. Remember, each of us is an experiment of one and what normally works well for most patients may be the wrong device for you.

Once you have settled in with the devices, it is imperative to bring the devices with you any time you buy a new pair of running shoes. If the orthotic device is important for you to stay healthy, then I recommend finding a shoe that works well with your orthotic as opposed to choosing the shoe first and seeing if the orthotic is compatible. The better running stores will have knowledge of which brands and models of shoe work best with custom orthotic devices. Not all runners will need or benefit from a foot orthotic device, but if chronic injuries are inhibiting your running, the devices might help to eliminate some or even all of your pain in conjunction with other treatments.

Chapter Two

Keeping Your Feet and Ankles Healthy (and Pretty!)

Running is tough on the feet. There are many seemingly minor issues that can get in the way of your training, at which point they are, by definition, not minor. In this chapter, we'll look at how to keep your feet and ankles functioning well and looking good.

Blisters

Blisters are caused by increased friction in an area and are commonly due to too much sweating or wetness in the socks or a boney prominence rubbing the wrong way in the shoe.

If blisters are a chronic problem and microfiber socks (see Chapter 1) aren't enough to prevent them, start by trying to cut down on the moisture in the sock and shoe. Spray your feet daily with an over-the-counter underarm antiperspirant spray. If you suffer from excessive sweating, talk with your doctor about prescription products designed for this problem. Soaking the feet in a diluted Burow's solution (an over-the-counter anti-bacterial product) can also cut down on the amount of sweat produced by the feet.

Try adding some lubricating gel or ointment such as Body Glide or Vaseline to the problem areas right before a run or workout. The ointments will cut down on the amount of friction and hopefully reduce the chance for blisters.

Once a blister develops, it's safe to puncture and drain the blister. Don't, however, completely de-roof the area by removing all the skin over the blister. You can sterilize a safety pin with rubbing alcohol, wipe the blister area clean with soap and water, and puncture the blister a couple of times to prevent the area from closing over and filling up again. Apply antibiotic ointment and make sure to keep the area clean and covered with a dry, sterile bandage when you go out for the day.

Keep an eye out for any redness or streaking that emanates from the area, as that could be the sign of a developing bacterial infection. If any pain or redness develops, immediately see your sports podiatrist for treatment, which could include an oral antibiotic. A staph infection will spread rapidly and could cause severe complications if not treated in a prudent fashion.

Black Nails

Keep your nails trimmed short. Longer nails have a great potential for trauma from a training run or race, which can lead to blood under the nail and sometimes losing the whole nail.

If the nail turns black after a run, a blood blister has formed under the nail and the nail will loosen from the skin underneath, which is called the nail bed. This can be a very painful injury; until the blister is drained it can hurt and throb constantly. A sterilized needle to drain the blister will relieve a lot of the pain and pressure from under the damaged nail. Use antibiotic ointment until the nail bed becomes less tender. A

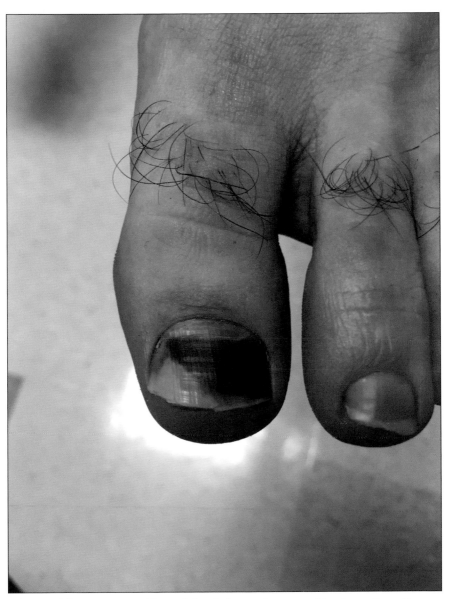

Black nail from trauma. If painful, a hole can be created in the nail to allow the blister to drain, which will relieve the pain.

Photo courtesy of Dr. Amol Saxena

few days after you drain the blister under the nail, the nail bed should become more comfortable.

Initially it's best to apply a bandage with some antibiotic ointment to keep the nail intact until it loosens naturally. A new nail begins to grow in immediately; the full growth of a big toe nail may take up to nine months. Proper fit of shoes, proper sock choice, and keeping the nails trimmed shorter can all help to prevent black toe nails from occurring. The size of the shoe should match the longest toe, which isn't always the big toe.

Ingrown Nails

Trim nails slightly curved across following the slightly rounded shape of the toe. Sometimes if you dig down into the corners of the nail an ingrown nail can be created, which might necessitate a visit to the podiatrist. For some, an ingrown nail is caused more by the underlying bone protruding up too much, causing a curved shape to the nail. Others are prone to them due to a genetic or inherited trait.

People with chronic, painful ingrown nails can have a procedure performed to permanently remove a portion of the nail. The procedure is called a matrixectomy. It's most commonly done as an in-office procedure with the use of a chemical such as phenol or sodium hydroxide to kill the nail matrix (the root of the nail where the nail forms). The procedure involves numbing the toe with a local anesthetic. While in college I had one side of my big toe nail corrected with phenol and ran eight miles the next day, so downtime is usually minimal.

Full healing will take a few weeks. The area will have some drainage during the two- to three-week healing period, but thcrc should never be another ingrown nail in the area if the procedure is successful.

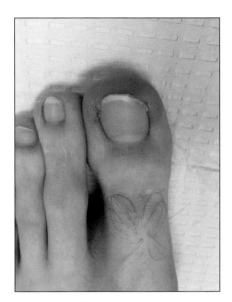

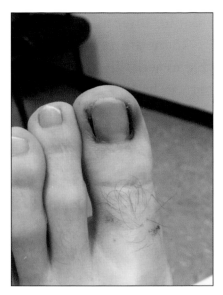

Ingrown nail. Note the curved nature of the nail growing in a horseshoe shape and causing pain with any pressure on the toe.

Ingrown nail after matrixectomy. The nail is removed from the sides and a chemical inactivates the nail root so that the sides never grow back.

Fungal Infection of Nail and Skin

Runners may sometimes have thicker-than-average nails, which are most often caused by repetitive trauma to the toes, but occasionally arc due to fungus invading the nail. Onychomycosis, or nail fungus, is a very difficult problem to resolve. If you get professional treatment, a culture of the nail to determine the causative organism can be performed. Depending on the culture result and the amount of nail affected, oral or topical medications can help cure the nail.

Terbinifine is the generic name for Lamisil, which is the most effective oral agent for nail fungus. Lamisil can cause elevated liver enzymes, among other possible complications, but with a success rate of up to 70 percent in some studies, it's the most effective treatment available. The patient takes one Lamisil pill a day for three months.

There are several prescription topical medications available as well. These are less effective than the oral medication but can be taken without the worry of side effects. The topical medications have to be used for a year continuously in order to be effective. There are three approved for use in the United States: Penlac (ciclopirox), Jublia (efinaconazole), and Keradyn (tavaborole). Those three medications are specially formulated to penetrate the nail; any other medication is not going to work very well.

For natural, over-the-counter remedies, Vick's VapoRub, tea tree oil, and Listerine all have antifungal properties, but in this condition the fungus resides under the nail, and most medications have difficulty penetrating the nail enough to be effective. An important fact to note is that even after successful treatment with an antifungal product that produces a normal-appearing nail, a subsequent nail can become infected with fungus again.

A final option for resistant cases of nail fungus is treatment in some podiatrists' offices with a laser. The laser treatment is typically not covered by insurance, so the patient incurs an out-of-pocket expense that can be several hundred dollars. Laser has been shown to be more effective than the topical medications and to have a similar success rate to oral Lamisil, but the cost and reinfection rate can make this treatment prohibitive for some.

Feet that are often in a moist environment may be susceptible to an athlete's foot infection, medically known as tinea

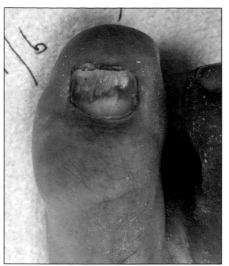 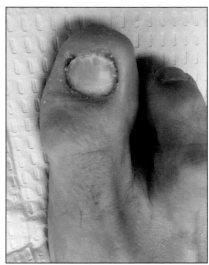

Runner's fungal nail before treatment.   Runner's nail after four months of treatment with Jublia.

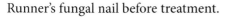

pedis, which is a fungal infection of the skin. If your feet have scaling skin that itches on the bottom of the foot and/or in between the toes, then you may have a tinea pedis infection. However, if the scaling is also in the arch of the foot, that's a sign of something else, as tinea pedis usually skips the arch of the foot.

Treatment must be done for at least a month, because new skin takes twenty-eight days to turn over. You can use an over-the-counter antifungal cream or get a prescription from your doctor. Make sure to dry very well between the toes—the tight spaces can allow fungus to thrive. (Fungus requires three things to be successful: darkness, warmth, and moisture.) A fungal infection can indirectly lead to a more serious bacterial infection, which can be created from scratching the fungal areas and developing an opening in the skin that serves as a point of entry for bacteria.

Kinesio Taping

Kinesio tape originated in Japan in the early 1970s and was invented by Dr. Kenso Kase, an American-trained chiropractor. Kase's theory was that the tape functions as a second skin to affect the sensory motor system, creating changes that allow tissue to heal. Kase thought that kinesio tape could help stimulate blood flow to an injured area due to the elasticity on the skin. There are some studies that show the benefits of kinesio tape, but many more disprove claims of improved strength and function from taping.

I find that kinesio tape is easier to self-apply than traditional athletic tape, can be worn in the shower, and definitely helps my injured patients. The many ways to utilize this tape in the foot and ankle are highlighted throughout this book. Perhaps the best aspect of this treatment is that if it doesn't work, there's no harm done.

Morton's Neuroma

A neuroma is a benign irritation of the nerves in the feet. They most commonly occur between the second and third toes, or between the third and fourth toes (known as the second and third interspaces, respectively). In 1876, T. G. Morton was the first to describe the nerve irritation being in the third interspace. The first surgical excision of a neuroma was described in 1883; to this day, surgery may involve removal of the thickened portion of this nerve.

Runners will experience shooting pain in the ball of the foot that sometimes radiates into the toes. The pain is increased with tighter shoes. Numbness will sometimes be felt in the affected toes. People with neuroma pain sometimes feel like their sock

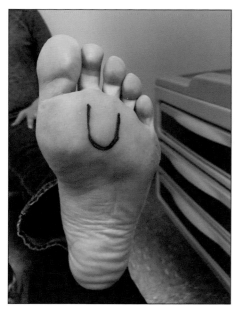

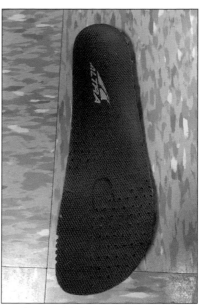

Neuroma pad marking the foot first. Use a felt-tip marker to mark around the painful area.

Mark on sock liner. Step on the sock liner to create a marker to show the proper spot for the padding.

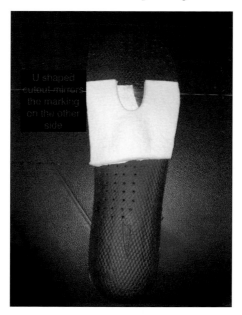

Pad on bottom of sock liner.

is bunched up under the toes or may feel like there's something under the ball of the foot causing an odd feeling under the toes.

The pain is often relieved when you take a tighter pair of shoes off your feet. Getting into a shoe with a wider toe box, such as the Altra brand, or a wider width shoe is one of the best initial treatments. A metatarsal pad can be placed on the sock liner of the running shoes to try to offload the pressure from the irritated nerve tissue, or a pad can be placed directly on the foot or added to an orthotic device.

When pain persists after changing shoes or adding padding, then a visit to your sports podiatrist is in order. The medical literature reveals that clinical examination is the best way to diagnose a neuroma. Feeling a "click" with compression of the foot

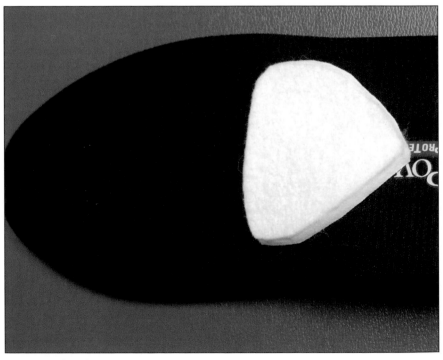

Metatarsal pad.

from side to side is known as a positive Mulder's sign. Feeling that click along with the nerve-type symptoms of numbness, burning, and shooting pain can confirm the diagnosis of a neuroma. MRIs and diagnostic ultrasound can also be performed to help confirm the diagnosis.

Custom padding or custom orthotic devices can work very well. Occasionally an injection of corticosteroid in the area can be very effective, but I caution against more than two or three injections per year in this area, and only with a low-dose steroid. Too many injections of cortisone in a short time can cause the ligaments around the toes in the area to degenerate and may lead to a deviated toe. A series of injections with a solution of 4 percent alcohol can be effective as well, but requires up to ten weekly injections, depending on how the foot responds. Shockwave therapy has also been utilized for this injury with some success.

If all conservative treatment fails, surgery should be considered. I expect runners to be able to return to activity around six weeks post-surgery depending on swelling and recovery. (See Chapter 8 for more on surgery.)

Skin Lesions

A build-up of excess skin may include several different types of lesions, from a simple callous to a painful corn or a wart. The body will react to any areas of increased pressure or stress by producing extra skin in the area, particularly around a boney prominence such as a hammer toe or a bone on the bottom of the foot, such as a metatarsal head. A corn can develop, and this extra skin goes deeper than the more superficial callus and can cause pain if the skin lesion is extending deeper.

A pumice stone can be used to grind down the excess skin in most cases, or padding, including gel or felt pads, can be used. Avoid any products that claim to help remove the corns—they contain acid, which can burn the normal skin if not placed directly on the thicker skin. Most podiatrists are skilled at debriding these lesions, and sometimes that's the only treatment required.

A wart is caused by a viral infection, the human papilloma virus, and is medically known as a verruca. When a verruca is located on the bottom of the foot, it's commonly referred to as a plantar wart. The difficulty in treating warts on the bottom of the foot is that the skin is thicker, leading the body to not recognizing the lesion is present and failing to mount an immune response to get rid of this often painful lesion. Warts are typically circular in shape. Small black dots may also be present; these represent small capillaries. The small blood vessels are coaxed to the area by the wart virus to use the body's vascular supply to help keep itself alive in a parasitic-type process. Blood vessels are often accompanied by nerve tissue, accounting for the pain from these lesions. Occasionally warts

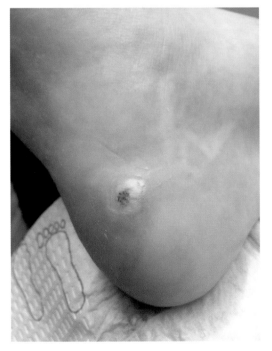

Classic plantar wart. Note the absence of skin lines within the wart.

Photo courtesy of Dr. Rob Conenello

will spontaneously resolve, but they can also multiply. If the wart is affecting your activity due to pain or if there are multiple warts, seek treatment.

Warts will respond better to early intervention; if left untreated, the lesions can spread throughout the whole body. If more than one wart is present, it's important to try to identify the original or "mother," as warts can spread to other parts of the body via a satellite process called the Koebner Phenomenon. Many times treatment of the mother wart can lead to all of the other lesions resolving. Treatment can be conservative, involving topical or oral medications, or surgical, to excise the lesion. Surgery on the bottom of the foot shouldn't be entered into lightly because if the excision extends too deep into the underlying tissue, scar tissue can form and be painful.

There are a lot of potential treatments listed in the literature. A single-trial study in *Family Practice Journal* several years ago found that covering the wart with duct tape helped to resolve the virus. But two subsequent studies found duct tape to be no better than a placebo. As with those for corns, over-the-counter wart products should be used with caution, because they contain acid that can burn normal skin if not placed in the exact location of the wart tissue.

In my office, I use a medication that combines three different medications: salicylic acid, podophyllin, and cantherone. Prescription topical medications can also help to resolve the warts. Adapalene 0.1 percent gel (Differin is the trade name) is a prescription topical acne medication that has been proven successful in the treatment of warts. Imiquimod (trade name is Aldara) is a topical agent that acts to enhance cell-mediated immunity. It's commonly used for treatment of squamous cell carcinoma and also can help to eliminate warts.

Oral medications can also help the immune system fight the wart virus to resolve the warts. Check with your physician before taking anything orally, especially if you are on other medications, to avoid any drug-to-drug interactions. Cimetadine (trade name is Tagamet) is a medication traditionally used for heartburn, but it can be a successful adjunct to treat plantar warts, taken at a dose of 25–40 mg/kg a day.

Oral vitamin A combined with zinc can also help the body eliminate these painful lesions. I recommend my patients who have resistant cases take 10,000 IUs of vitamin A and 15 mg of zinc twice a day. Topical vitamin A can also be applied to the wart in between visits to the podiatry office.

Stone Bruise (Metatarsalgia)

A stone bruise is the lay term for pain under the ball of the foot or metatarsal heads. Medically known as metatarsalgia, this term can encompass several different diagnoses. Inflammation of the joint is the simplest form. If you recall landing on a rock or a similar hard object, then a bruise should resolve within a week or so by using ice, avoiding being barefoot, and adding some padding behind the area where it hurts.

A more serious form of metatarsalgia can occur if the plantar plate is damaged. The plantar plate is a small piece of cartilage-like material located under the metatarsal-phalangeal joint (MPJ) that provides stability to the joint. If a small tear occurs, then the affected toe may elevate above the other digits and lead to significant pain under the MPJ, with swelling over the top of the joint often noted. Conservative treatment can include taping the affected toe down to relieve the pressure from the area. This joint can function like a see-saw—as the toe goes up in the

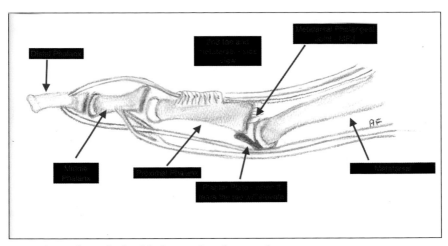

A toe from the side, highlighting the plantar plate.

Drawing by Annemarie Fullem, PT

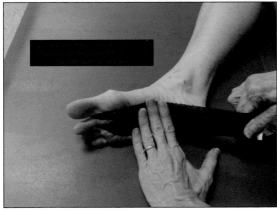

Patient with elevated toe due to tear of plantar plate.

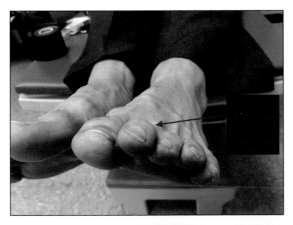

Taping for plantar plate tear.

air more, there will be more pressure on the bottom of the joint. A surgical shoe can be a good adjunct. In severe cases surgery may be required.

Ankle Sprains

Ankle sprains are the most common sports injury but not as prevalent in runners. The most common ankle sprain is an inversion-type sprain, in which you roll over the outside of the foot and injure the lateral structures of the ankle. There are three ligaments that could be damaged in an ankle sprain. The first ligament that typically suffers damage is the anterior talo-fibular ligament (ATFL). In a simple lateral sprain it's often the only ligament damaged. The calcaneal-fibular ligament (CFL) is the second ligament to undergo damage in a lateral sprain, and is often hurt in conjunction with injury to the ATFL.

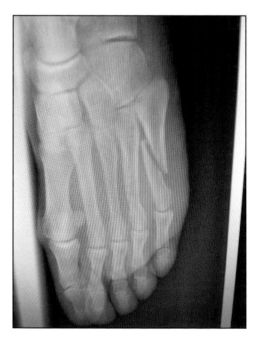

After an ankle sprain an X-ray is very important to obtain, because if a fracture occurs during the injury the treatment protocol changes. Make sure that the foot is X-rayed, because the fifth metatarsal can be injured as well.

At left is a photo of an X-ray of a runner who rolled his ankle on a trail

Fracture of fifth metatarsal of a runner with ankle sprain.

run. The ankle was slightly sprained but the foot required surgical correction for the fracture of the fifth metatarsal.

If a fracture is noted in any other areas then a removable cast boot may be required for two to four weeks. Keep in mind that any time the foot or leg is immobilized there will be atrophy of the surrounding muscles, and strengthening and proprioception will be required before a return to activity. It's preferable to not immobilize the foot and leg completely if possible because studies have shown that this leads to scar tissue formation in addition to inhibiting proprioception.

Ankle sprains are assigned Grades 1 to 3, based on the severity of the injury. Grade 1 is a minor strain with no tearing of the ligaments. There may be some pain and swelling but there's usually not any associated bruising. It will typically heal within a month. Grade 2 is a partial tear, usually of the ATFL first, followed by the CFL. Grade 3 is a complete tear of one or more of the ligaments.

Eversion ankle sprains, which cause damage to the medial malleolus or inside of the foot, are less common, with damage to the deltoid ligament occurring. Make sure to note if there are areas of pain and swelling other than around the ankle bones.

Range-of-motion exercises should be started as soon as pain subsides enough. A good start is to draw the letters of the alphabet with your foot. Exercises with a Thera-band are a good next step for rehab to strengthen the foot against resistance until weight-bearing exercises can be instituted. Balance and restoring the proper function of the tendons must be performed as soon as possible. Ideally, proprioception will be restored before considering return to activity. (More detail on balance and proprioception exercises found in Chapter 6.) Surgery is rarely

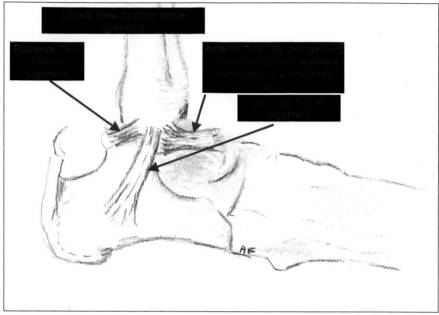

Ankle ligaments. The lateral ankle ligaments are highlighted.
Drawing by Annemarie Fullem, PT

required for an ankle sprain regardless of the severity of the ligament damage.

Talar Dome Injury

The talus bone sits at the top of the foot and helps to form the ankle joint along with the end of the tibia. This bone is covered with cartilage, which is a smooth surface that can be damaged in a severe ankle sprain. If pain persists inside the ankle joint after a sprain, then an MRI or CT scan may be required to inspect the cartilage on top of the talus. If the talus suffers damage, it's known as a talar dome lesion and may require surgical intervention, which in a lot of cases can be performed arthroscopically.

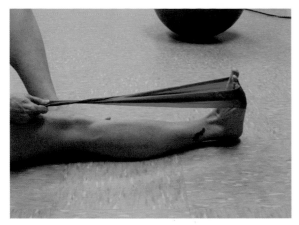

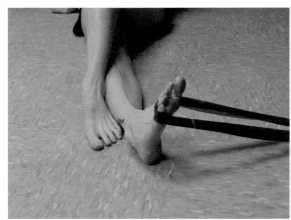

Using a Thera-Band, you can begin strengthening within a few days after a sprain.

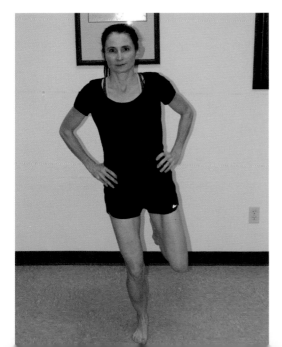

Balancing on one foot.

Midfoot Sprain (Lisfranc's Injury)

These injuries are less common in the runner, but stepping in a hole or twisting the forefoot can lead to an injury in the middle of the foot. The tarso-metatarsal joint is known as Lisfranc's joint; the other joints are considered midfoot joints. Pain and swelling may be noted on the top of the foot. An X-ray can sometimes reveal small avulsion-type fractures. A Lisfranc's injury can be detected with a clinical exam, in which moving the first and second metatarsals in different directions will cause pain. X-rays can sometimes detect a small fracture of the base of the second metatarsal caused by the ligament being overstressed and pulling a piece of bone away. (This is known as the "Fleck" sign.)

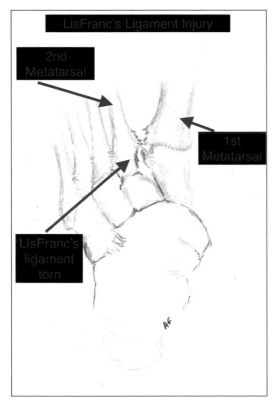

Radiographs will reveal a wider gap between the base of the first and second metatarsal bases. If the gap is greater than 2 mm, surgery is indicated, which involves placing a screw or sometimes a new technique known as a "tightrope" procedure can be performed.

Lisfranc injury. Note the separation of the first metatarsal from the second metatarsal.

Drawing by Annemarie Fullem, PT

The latter uses suture material to close the gap and realign the foot.

Sinus Tarsi Syndrome

The sinus tarsi is a canal between the talus and calcaneus. This can be a difficult injury to detect, as the pain felt may be nondescript. A simple ankle sprain or instability of the foot can lead to inflammation of the nerve in this area. Pain will be felt over the front lateral aspect of the foot.

The injury is difficult to treat at home. I've found that an injection of corticosteroid and local anesthetic can work very well. In a foot that exhibits excessive motion, a custom orthotic can be considered if the injection doesn't resolve the pain or if the pain keeps recurring. Surgery should be an absolute last resort and shouldn't be considered if an injection of local

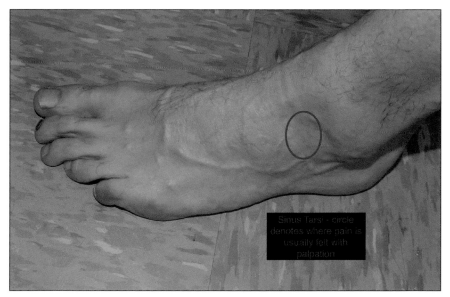

Photo highlighting the sinus tarsi area.

anesthetic doesn't resolve the pain immediately after the shot is performed.

Keeping the feet looking good can be a difficult task for a runner. Any painful swelling in the foot that lasts longer than a few days should result in a visit to your sports podiatrist. Don't let injuries progress to the chronic stage before seeking treatment—ignoring a problem and hoping it will go away is never the best course of action in the case of a runner's feet.

Chapter Three

Plantar Fasciitis and Other Types of Heel Pain

It's estimated that there are more than three million doctor visits a year in the United States for heel pain alone. The most common cause of heel pain in runners is plantar fasciitis, but there are a number of different causes of pain in the heel besides the plantar fascia, with the location and type of pain offering clues as to the possible diagnosis. Some of the different diagnoses besides plantar fasciitis include nerve problems, stress fractures of the heel bone, and a tear or complete rupture of the fascia.

In this chapter we'll look at the most common running injuries to the heel, starting with the biggie, plantar fasciitis.

Plantar Fasciitis

Let's begin by using the proper terminology. In plantar fasciitis, the fascia isn't really inflamed. In one study, tissue samples from surgery to release the fascia were analyzed and failed to demonstrate any inflammatory cells under a microscope. "Plantar fasciosis," indicating degeneration rather than inflammation of tissue, may be a better term as the fascia, in a similar fashion

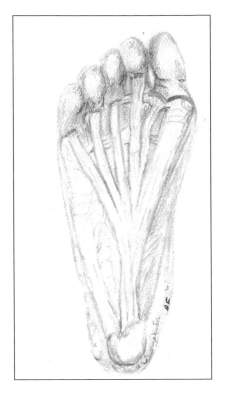

The first layer under the skin of the bottom of the foot, highlighting the plantar fascia.

Drawing by Annemarie Fullem, PT

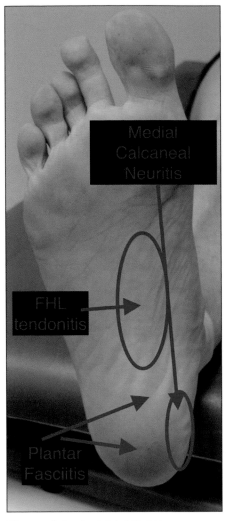

Photo of the foot, highlighting the different areas of the heel that correspond to different diagnoses.

to tendons, begins to degenerate when injured for an extended period of time. Usually, an injury to the plantar fascia lasting longer than a month is entering a chronic stage. For the sake of familiarity, we'll use the terms "plantar fasciitis" and "plantar fasciosis" interchangeably.

Fascia is similar to a ligament. It's a rope-like structure with very little elasticity, the lack of which enables it to help support the area it surrounds. Consider it the infrastructure of the body. "Plantar" means "bottom of the foot." The plantar fascia begins at the heel bone and shares some fibers with the end of the Achilles tendon. The structure then runs the length of the foot and splits near the toes into slips under each digit. The main attachment is at the plantar medial tubercle of the calcaneus (heel bone); that's one of the three common places that pain from fasciosis occurs. Directly under the middle of the bottom of the calcaneus is the second most common area for plantar fascia pain. Less commonly, there can be pain along the outside of the bottom of the foot behind the fifth metatarsal (referred to as the lateral band of the plantar fascia). If the pain is in other than those three spots, then it's probably not plantar fasciosis.

Plantar fasciitis typically causes significant pain when you take your first steps in the morning and after sitting; this is known as post-static dyskinesia. The longer the process progresses, the more painful the foot will become beyond the initial steps until there is constant pain. People who have to stand a lot are susceptible, as feet are much better made for walking than standing. As with most injuries, early treatment significantly increases the chances for successful treatment. An important fact to note is that fascia doesn't have much elasticity and thus is unable to be stretched. Instead, self-treatment should involve stretching the calf muscles, as the calf muscles become the Achilles, and by loosening the Achilles there will be less stress on the fascia.

I recommend the simple wall stretch. Stretch each leg individually for thirty seconds, and repeat five times, three different times during the day. The stretch should be felt in the calf muscles, not in the heel or Achilles tendon.

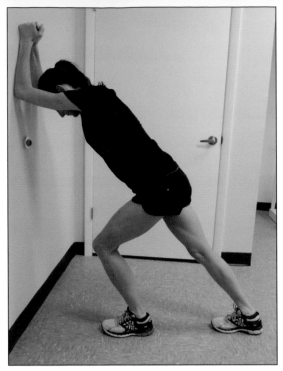

How to properly stretch the calf when experiencing plantar fascia pain. Keep the back foot flat on the ground, knee straight and lean in until a good stretch is felt in the calf. There should be no pain.

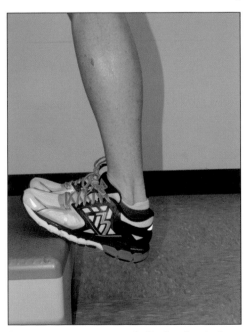

Improper way to stretch for heel pain by hanging off a step. Doing so can cause more traction and pain on the fascia.

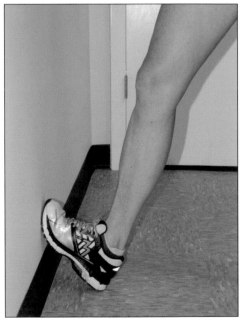

Another improper way to stretch the fascia, by putting your toes up against a wall. Doing so will cause too much tension in the foot.

Another stretch that involves pulling the toes back and massaging the fascia has shown good results in two medical articles.

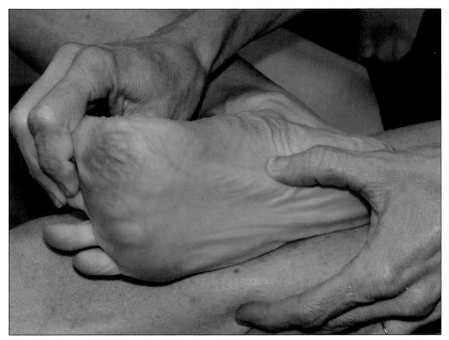

Pull the toes back and use your thumb to massage along the fascia. Hold for 10 seconds and repeat 10 times, several times a day.

Icing with a frozen water bottle is one of the better ways to alleviate plantar fascia pain. Roll your arch and heel over the frozen bottle every night for 10 to 15 minutes. I don't find standard anti-inflammatories, such as ibuprofen, to be very effective for this injury, because there's not an inflammatory process happening in the fascia. Anti-inflammatories might provide some pain relief but they aren't worth the potential side effects, which can be significant. John Mortimer was a high school national champion and many-time All-American distance runner at the University of Michigan. John developed kidney disease during

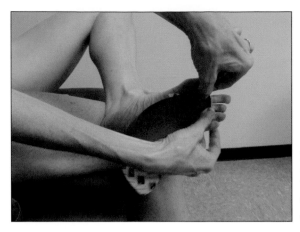

Applying kinesio tape for heel pain: Start behind the toes with no tension on the first 1" of tape applied.

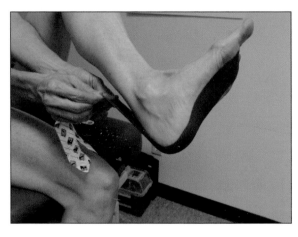

Put the tape under a stretch as you attach to the skin and continue up the back of heel over the Achilles. End with no tension on the last 1" of tape.

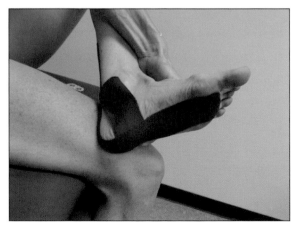

Finally, a second strip can be placed across the painful area. Tear the tape in the middle, apply tension and lay the tape down on each side with no tension.

his running career, and the disease was thought to be directly related to his frequent use of over-the-counter anti-inflammatories. Use of medications such as Aleve and Motrin may also mask the symptoms, leading to a more serious injury.

Some people claim that running in barefoot-type shoes can cure plantar fasciitis. There is zero medical evidence to support this claim. I believe that this injury will respond better when the foot is well supported until the pain subsides. We discussed barefoot/minimalist running in Chapter 1. Patients with plantar fasciosis almost always feel better when taped.

One of my patients was running over 100 miles per week, which makes it difficult for any injury, let alone plantar fasciosis, to heal. This patient was resistant to the idea of custom orthotic devices and he was mostly pain-free while running with tape on his arch. He taped his foot pre-run for almost two years, and during this time ran 2:16 at the Boston Marathon! Medical studies show that tape provides proprioceptive feedback to the body, thereby making the body perceive that the area taped is being supported. There's no need to worry that you'll become dependent on the tape. An arch support can often relieve some of the pain by reducing some of the stress on the fascia. There are several well-made over-the-counter inserts. The device shouldn't be too rigid; if it is, it might be too uncomfortable to run in. Walk around in the devices to make sure they're a good fit before running in them. Another option is a soft heel cup, which are sometimes made out of silicone or a similar foam-type material.

A night splint may help the injury improve, particularly with the first-steps pain. The device is worn while sleeping and places the foot in a position that helps to relieve some of the pain and helps to stretch the plantar fascia during the night. There are

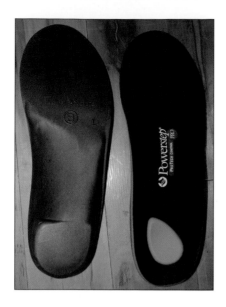

An over-the-counter type of insert.

two main types, sock types and more rigid devices with plastic support. People who have difficulty sleeping may not respond well to night splints.

As is the case with most injuries, check your training shoes to make sure they're not overly worn. If you have several pairs in your rotation, write the date you first wear your new shoes on the midsole and make a note in your training log. Doing so makes it easy to track the amount of mileage on a pair of shoes.

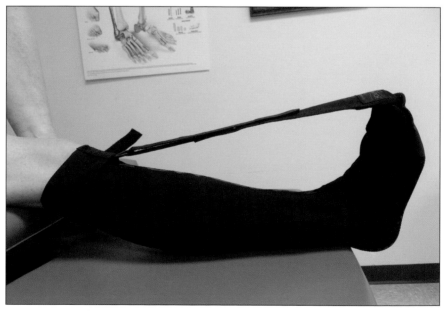

A sock-type night splint. Don't pull the front strap too much or the toes will be uncomfortable.

When to See a Podiatrist

Heel pain that lingers longer than several weeks should be investigated by your sports podiatrist. An X-ray is often performed, but don't put a lot of stock in the presence or absence of a heel spur seen on an X-ray. The spur is not pointing down and is deeply embedded in the muscles of the foot, and typically not involved in causing plantar fasciosis.

A proper exam should involve a physical exam, including a gait exam and manual muscle testing. You can help the doctor make the diagnosis by providing as much information as possible about any changes in training, including the amount of mileage on a pair of shoes, the introduction of faster or longer training, and any stresses in the rest of your life.

Treatment will be guided by how long the symptoms have been present and how quickly the patient wants to return to running. For example, a patient who is two weeks out from a goal race may require a more aggressive treatment plan. In those cases, I sometimes offer an injection into the area consisting of a mixture of a local anesthetic and a corticosteroid (the best known one of which is cortisone).

The medical evidence reveals that corticosteroid injections are effective in the short term, but not as effective for long-term results. I find that an injection works better when it's given close to the onset of pain. I inject directly into the bottom of the foot after identifying the area that hurts the most with palpation. Injecting under the guidance of diagnostic ultrasound is the most accurate method for proper placement of the needle, but is not typically necessary for an injection in this area, because when you inject from the bottom you avoid damage by the needle to any vital structures such as the nerve.

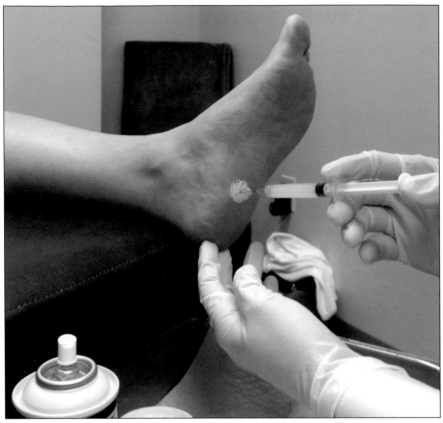

Injection of cortisone for plantar fascia pain.

It's very important to note that an injection of cortisone can make the plantar fascia more susceptible to a tear or rupture of the fascia. That said, in twenty-five years of treating heel pain in runners I have injected the plantar fascia area of more than one thousand patients and to my knowledge only one patient ruptured their plantar fascia during a run. We'll look more at plantar fascia tears later in this chapter.

Extracorporeal Shockwave Therapy is one of the best treatments for a long-term cure and is considered the gold standard for treatment of heel pain. EPAT (Extracorporeal Pulse

Activated Treatment) is a form of shockwave therapy that's available in office.

The treatment typically involves three to five treatments spaced a week or two apart. Shockwave therapy stimulates the body to produce new blood vessels to help the tissue heal. The initial forms of shockwave fifteen years ago required local anesthesia due to the severe pain associated with the treatment, and the units were large and brought to the office by an outside company. Newer units are smaller and almost never require anesthesia. The best aspects of the more modern machines are that the athlete can continue to train during the treatment, and the therapy doesn't cause harm. Insurance companies mostly consider the treatment experimental despite the voluminous amount of medical evidence in peer-reviewed literature that shows shockwave therapy to be the gold standard of conservative treatment for heel pain.

If patients have used over-the-counter inserts and are still experiencing symptoms, then a custom orthotic device can work very well. There are many options when choosing an orthotic device, including style, material, and additional options such as posting of the device to add more support in certain areas. (Orthotic therapy is covered in more detail in Chapter 1.)

Most custom orthotic devices will work well in running shoes; occasionally, the devices can also be fabricated for racing flats and spikes. One of the most important aspects of the device is how it's fabricated. I prefer to use plaster and perform the casting myself, as opposed to some offices that have medical assistants take the impression. Foam boxes and computer scanners are unable to capture the foot or certain deformities as well as plaster and may lead to a less-effective device.

The plaster impression is often then sent to an orthotic lab to create the device. The two most important aspects of custom orthotic devices is that they should reduce or prevent the symptoms of an injury and be comfortable. Choice of device material and posting should be based on several factors, including injury history, foot type, and the patient's prior experience with inserts. If a patient has used a more rigid orthotic device in the past and was unable to tolerate the hardness of the foot insert, then I typically create a softer, more flexible device, and vice versa. I create devices using several different labs and materials, including graphite, polyethylene, and other plastics, cork, and foam materials such as PORON and Spenco.

When Heel Pain Isn't Plantar Fasciitis

In 2001, Weldon Johnson, elite runner and co-founder of the popular running website LetsRun.com, had a huge career

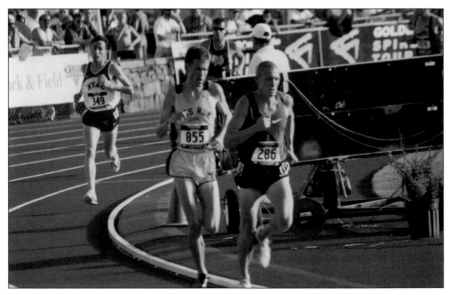

Weldon Johnson (#855) finishing fourth in the 2001 U.S. 10,000-meter championships.

breakthrough, finishing fourth at the US championships in the 10,000 meters and running 28:10 for the distance. That autumn, however, he developed heel pain and was treated by several physicians and therapists with no success.

I met Weldon at a track meet in Boston, and he explained that his symptoms didn't include more pain with his first steps in the morning and was localized to the inside of his heel. The presentation was more similar to medial calcaneal neuritis, an inflammation of the nerve. The location is close to the same spot as plantar fasciosis but doesn't respond well to rest or the usual treatments that help fasciosis improve.

One treatment that can be very effective for this injury is a local injection. I typically use 1 cc of Marcaine (a long-acting local anesthetic), 4 mg of Dexamethasone Phosphate (a soluble corticosteroid), and 3 mg of Celestone (an insoluble

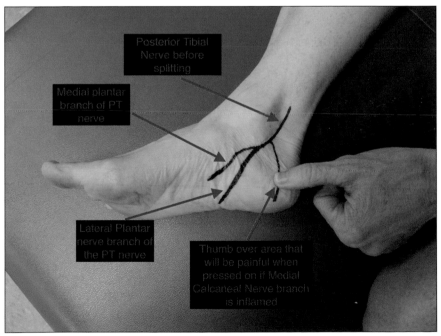

Depiction of the nerve branches of the heel.

corticosteroid, which is longer acting than a soluble ste-roid). I injected Weldon's medial calcaneal nerve area and he improved significantly. Several weeks later a second injection in the same spot resolved all his pain there permanently, and in 2003 Weldon improved his 10K PR to 28:06 while finishing fourth in the national championships and beating four-time US Olympian Abdi Abdriraham, among others.

The medial calcaneal nerve is a branch of the lateral plantar nerve as it enters the foot. It will cause heel pain that mimics plantar fasciitis in some ways but it definitely will not feel bet-ter taped, and the pain does not subside after initial discomfort and isn't necessarily worse with first steps. Rest, ice, and keep-ing pressure off the area should all be parts of the treatment plan. Sometimes a firm or hard orthotic device can exacerbate the symptoms, so an insert is not always the best option for this injury.

Plantar Fascia Rupture

In 1983, I was running a 2-mile race on Bucknell's indoor track. The good: I ran 8:59, my first time under 9:00. The bad: I tore my plantar fascia coming off the last turn. I was treated initially by an orthopedist, was told it was plantar fasciitis, and given an injection; I was provided with no other advice. I later saw a podiatrist, who added rigid custom orthotic devices (which may not have been the best choice for my high-arched foot type) and stretching to the treatment as well as a second injec-tion. The podiatrist also failed to recognize it was a tear, as, in retrospect, I felt a pop in my foot and after finishing the race my foot became more and more painful until I had difficulty stand-ing on it the next day.

Ruptures of the plantar fascia aren't always abrupt or complete, but if the pain is farther away from the heel and there's accompanying bruising or swelling, then a rupture may have occurred. I advise my patients that, as reported in an article I co-authored in the *American Journal of Sports Medicine* in 2004, this injury can take an average of nine weeks before you can return to activity. Often after a tear of the fascia is healed, the patient will no longer experience plantar fasciitis. The final treatment for plantar fasciitis sometimes involves surgery to release the fascia, so a patient who sustains a plantar fascia tear has essentially performed their own surgery.

Treatment of a tear initially involves immobilization in a walking boot for one to three weeks. If there's pain when walking in the boot, then crutches or a knee walker should be used until you can walk pain-free in the boot. Physical therapy can

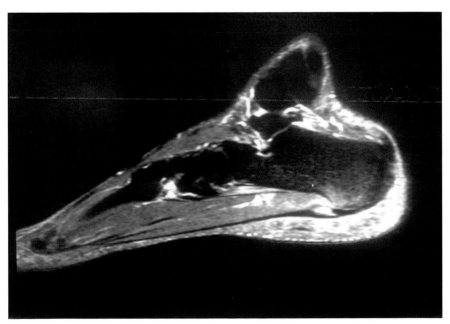

MRI of the foot showing a partial tear of the plantar fascia.

be initiated with a focus on eliminating the rest of the pain, improving flexibility and strengthening the foot and leg. Taping or an arch support can also be used to allow the tissue to heal better. MRI and diagnostic ultrasound are two great modalities to help make an accurate diagnosis. Above is an MRI of an athlete with a partial tear of the fascia.

Tarsal Tunnel Syndrome

The tarsal tunnel is analogous to the carpal tunnel in the wrist. This area is located behind and around the medial malleolus, which is the inside ankle bone that is the end of the tibia bone. Pain will sometimes mimic plantar fasciosis or medial calcaneal neuritis, because the nerve sends signals to the same area where plantar fasciitis causes pain, but is much more resistant to treatment, and finding the cause can prove difficult.

Tarsal tunnel syndrome (TTS) is an entrapment of the posterior tibial nerve, which runs behind the medial malleolus along with the tendons and blood vessels into the bottom of the foot. The covering of this tunnel is the flexor retinaculum, which is a ligament that's also attached to the plantar fascia. Tension on the plantar fascia can lead to more stress in this area.

There are three tendons entering the foot after starting as muscles in the leg: the posterior tibial tendon, the flexor hallucis longus tendon, and the flexor digitorum longus tendon. Each tendon is separated by ligamentous structures known as the septa. The septa create channels to allow the structures in the leg to transition into the foot. The septa also form the walls of the tarsal tunnel, with the three tendons forming the floor of the tunnel.

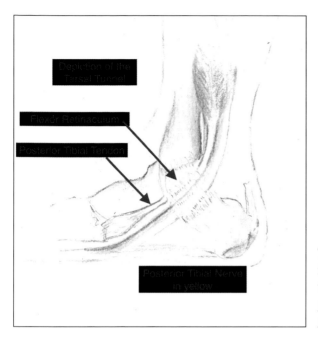

The medial side of the foot, highlighting the tarsal tunnel.

Drawing by Annemarie Fullem, PT.

There are several reasons for TTS, including the existence of a soft tissue mass such as a ganglion; inflammation or tendinosis causing thickening or swelling; and a varicosity of the vein that takes up too much space in the area, leading to irritation of the nerve. The biomechanics of the foot can also predispose one to this injury. The fascia covering the abductor hallucis muscle belly can also lead to nerve compression if the muscle becomes hypertrophied.

In addition to heel pain, TTS can cause radiating pain similar to an electric-shock-type feeling that can shoot down the bottom of the foot into the toes. There may also be areas of numbness in the heel or arch related to the nerve not functioning properly. If the nerve has been compressed for a long period of time, then sensory loss and weakness of the muscles in the feet may result in atrophy and the formation of hammertoes.

If you have a history of back pain, this should also be investigated as a possible cause. Spinal nerve roots L4, L5, S1, and S2 form the sciatic nerve and supply most of the innervation to the foot and leg. It's imperative to rule out radiculopathy—pain in the foot or leg that originates in the back at the area where the nerves leave the back—as the cause, especially if surgery is being considered.

One test for TTS is to tap on the inside of the ankle over the tarsal tunnel area. If this elicits tingling down into the foot or heel, this is known as a positive Tinnel's sign and indicates a possible diagnosis of TTS. An MRI should be performed to rule out any soft tissue masses or other possible causes.

Nerve conduction velocity (NCV) is a test that a neurologist can perform. An NCV test involves placing needles into the foot and leg to measure the speed of the nerve after it's stimulated. A comparison is then made between the affected and unaffected limb, and if there is a difference of greater than 50 percent, that can help make the diagnosis. It should be noted that the NCV test is dependent on the expertise of the examiner, and false negative findings are not uncommon.

A local nerve block can be performed with some corticosteroid added to help make a diagnosis. If there's complete pain relief after an injection containing local anesthetic, then that can help to narrow the diagnosis, pointing towards TTS as being the cause. Other conservative treatments include custom orthotic devices and physical therapy.

In cases resistant to conservative therapy, surgery can be considered. In the simplest cases, this involves cutting all the ligaments and fascia covering the posterior tibial nerve. The success rate varies with reports in the medical literature, but a range of 75 percent to 91 percent is reported in the most recent studies on the topic. Surgery is typically more successful in eliminating symptoms if the cause is a soft tissue mass or other space-occupying lesion.

Haglund's Deformity/Posterior Heel Spur

Pain in the back of the heel may be due to a boney prominence in the back of the heel bone known as a Haglund's deformity, or it can be due to a spur protruding off the back of the calcaneus into the insertion of the Achilles tendon. The tendon will often be irritated by the interface of the back of the heel with the running shoe. A hard heel counter can aggravate any boney prominence in the back of the heel and make running difficult. A bursitis may also develop in the area, leading to the appearance of swelling.

Stretching the calf muscles, icing, and removing anything that's irritating the back of the heel in the shoe are all good first lines of treatment. Additionally, adding a heel lift may help to reduce some of the pain. If you do so, place a silicone heel cup into both shoes so as not to cause a limb-length discrepancy.

Note that this area doesn't typically respond well to strengthening or direct stretching of the area. Massage should also be avoided over the back of the heel bone. Any stretch should be felt higher up in the calf. Attempts to stretch by hanging off a step or even bending the back leg to feel more of a stretch in the lower Achilles should be avoided, as this can cause more pain and prolong the course of the injury.

In the presence of a large spur or bump in the back of the heel, it's possible to alleviate some of the pain by cutting the heel

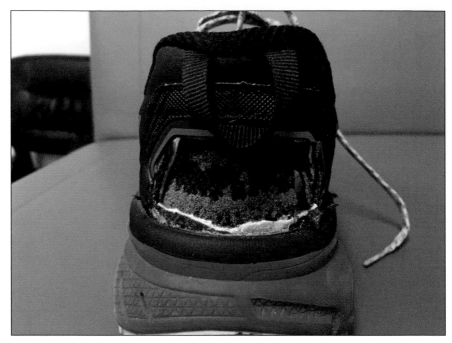

A cutout of the heel counter in the back of the shoe to alleviate pain from a bone spur in the back of the heel.

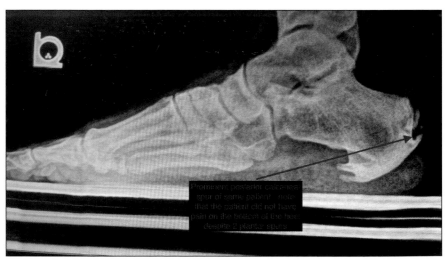

X-ray of severe spurring in the back of the heel bone.

counter out or switching to a shoe without a firm heel counter, such as the Nike Free series. Resistant cases may require surgical intervention, but I would always recommend the use of shockwave therapy before considering surgery. Surgical management for this injury is covered in detail in Chapter 8.

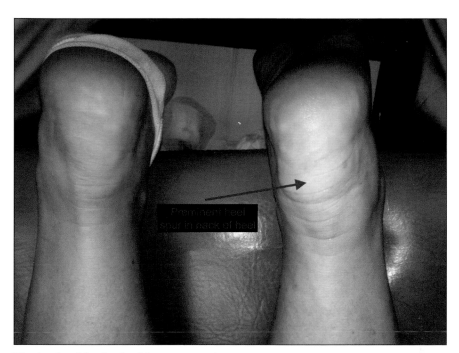

The back of the heel of the same patient.

Stress Fracture of the Calcaneus

If your heel pain isn't responding to treatments, then further investigation is necessary and a stress fracture of the calcaneus may need to be ruled out. This injury is discussed in more detail in Chapter 5. A stress fracture can mimic the pain of a severe case of plantar fasciitis. Some of the symptoms will be different in a fracture as the pain isn't worse during your first steps, as in plantar fasciitis, but rather worsens during the day.

Additionally, the pain will not be relieved by taping or arch support.

The proper diagnosis and treatment is often based on the subjective symptoms of the runner. Keep track of where it hurts the most, what time of day it hurts the most, what aggravates the pain and what makes it feel better. Try to track the types of symptoms, such as sharp pain, dull ache, numbness, tingling, or radiating pain. The more information that you provide to the sports medicine specialist, then the greater your chances of having successful treatment. If the pain isn't worse with your first steps in the morning and after sitting, or if some of the treatments that normally help plantar fasciitis don't help, then it's important to investigate the other causes of heel pain besides plantar fasciitis.

Chapter Four
Tendon Injuries

Tendons serve as the pulley mechanism for our skeletal system. They extend from the end of a muscle to provide the attachment to bone, occasionally by taking sharp turns around boney prominences. When a tendon is injured we commonly refer to it as tendonitis.

The term "tendonitis" connotes inflammation, but this is only true within the first two weeks of the tendon injury. A medical study showed that, under microscopic examination, an injured Achilles tendon showed no inflammatory cells within the tendon; instead, there was degeneration, leading to the term "tendinosis" as a more apt, all-encompassing word. This change of perspective has led to a greater understanding in the treatment of tendon injuries. Still, the terms "tendonitis" and "tendinosis" are often used interchangeably.

In this chapter, we'll look at the most common tendon injuries, including what most runners call shin splints.

Achilles Tendinosis

The Achilles tendon is the largest tendon in the body. Injury to it is one of the more difficult conditions to treat in a runner.

There are only a few injuries that might lead me as a sports medicine podiatrist to advise runners that they might have to take time off, or at a minimum cross train and cut back on running. Achilles tendinopathy is one of those diagnoses.

The Achilles tendon is formed from three calf muscles: the medial and lateral heads of the gastrocnemius muscle and the soleus muscle, which is beneath those two muscles. The gastrocnemius muscles start above the knee, while the soleus originates below the knee. The three muscles then merge in the lower half of the calf and form the Achilles tendon. This is an important fact to note when stretching this group. When the knee is locked during a calf stretch, it isolates the gastrocs; bending the knee helps to better stretch the soleus.

Anatomically, the Achilles differs from all the other tendons in the body because of its surrounding sheath. Most tendons are surrounded by a synovial sheath, which provides a layer of protection to the tendon and produces synovial fluid to help the tendon glide smoothly. The Achilles is covered by paratenon, which is a fibrous layer of tissue that provides the blood supply to the tendon and is thicker than the sheath covering other tendons.

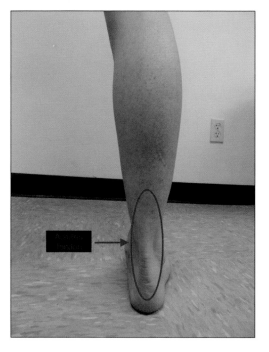

Back of the leg, highlighting the Achilles.

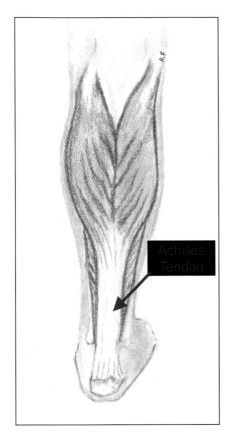

The Achilles.
Drawing by Annemarie Fullem, PT

The Achilles tendon serves to decelerate the forward motion of the leg when the foot initially contacts the ground. Then the load is gradually increased on the tendon until you reach toe-off. At toe-off (propulsion) up to six to eight times of your body weight is transmitted though the tendon. The tendon also serves to help resupinate the foot to prepare for the next foot strike. If the foot is pronating a significant amount, then the Achilles has to work harder to compensate for the excessive inward motion.

Pain in the Achilles can occur in three sites: mid substance of the tendon, at the insertion, and along the paratenon. Often the mid substance tendinosis will have an associated visible lump (see the photo on the next page). This type is characterized by more pain with initial activity that warms up and feels better during activity in the initial stages; however, as degeneration progresses, there will be pain with each step. Paratendinosis, which is thickening and damage of the paratenon, leads to scarring of the paratenon to the Achilles tendon, which prevents the normal gliding of the tendon. This form of Achilles injury leads

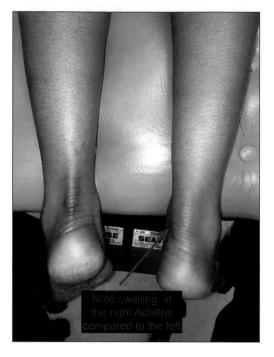

Achilles with tendinosis. Note the swelling.

to more pain with activity. Insertional Achilles issues are often associated with a prominent back-of-the-heel bone or spur. If the top part of the back of the calcaneus is more pronounced, this is known as a Haglund's deformity. (See Chapter 3 for more on that condition.)

The most common cause of Achilles tendinopathy is overuse. Tendons will typically not get injured until they're fatigued. Another very important cause is weakness of the core muscles, in particular the gluteal (butt) muscles. Other contributing factors could include changes in training terrain, changing shoes, training in the morning when the muscles and tendons are less pliable and warm, increases in training intensity, and adding speed work or hill work.

Three miscellaneous causes of tendon pathology include prior use of oral steroids, the use of statin drugs for high cholesterol, and the antibiotic class known as quinolones, which includes the commonly prescribed drugs Cipro (ciprofloxacin) and Levaquin (levofloxacin). The Achilles tendon should never be injected directly with any corticosteroid; doing so greatly increases the chances of rupture. Ryan Howard, a

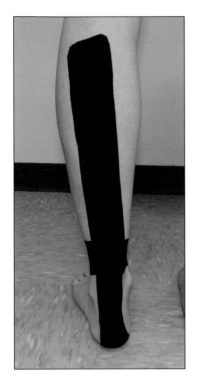

Kinesio tape applied for Achilles tendinosis. Start at the ball of the foot with no tension, then put the tape under about 50 percent of a stretch around the back of the heel and end above the Achilles on the calf muscle. A second strip can be placed perpendicular to the base strip over the area where there's pain and swelling.

baseball player for the Philadelphia Phillies, was injected twice into his Achilles, and a few weeks later he ruptured the tendon in a game.

The most important aspect of treating this injury is early intervention and treatment. Rest is sometimes necessary for this injury to improve. As is the case in the beginning of most injuries, it will warm up initially at the start of a run and the run can be completed pain-free. My rule of thumb is that if there is swelling, burning, and/or pain, then you should take some time off from running until the swelling subsides and you can run without pain. Taping can help with symptoms. Kinesio tape can be applied easily at home.

I recommend static calf stretching for five minutes, three times a day. Hold the stretch for thirty seconds at a time with short breaks. There are other methods of stretching that may be just as effective (PNF, contract/relax, and the active isolated method, popularized by sports medicine experts Jim and Phil Wharton), but static stretching is very safe. It's crucial to keep the foot flat on the ground because the gastroc-soleus muscle group can't stretch unless it's relaxed. Runners should

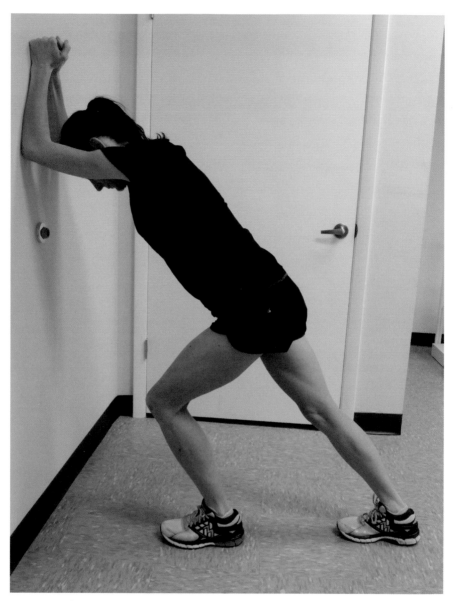

Proper calf stretch. Note the back foot completely on the ground. Lean in until a stretch is felt and hold for 30 seconds. Repeat 3-5 times three times during the day.

never hang off a step or curb and feel the stretch in the tendon itself. Also, stretching should never cause pain.

You can combine icing and stretching when seated with your foot in a bucket. Fill the bucket with ice cubes and water, and gently stretch the tendon with your toes up on the wall of the bucket. It's my opinion that anti-inflammatories such as ibuprofen (Advil, Motrin) or naproxen (Aleve) shouldn't be used for more than a few days, because they won't help a degenerated tendon and may mask the pain. A degenerated tendon is more susceptible to rupturing or tearing.

Massage is another excellent treatment, but it should be performed in different locations of the tendon, depending on whether you have tendinosis or paratenodosis. When there's more diffuse swelling and you can feel crepitus (a crunchy feeling), then this is more closely associated with inflammation of the paratenon. When swelling is more focal (localized) and lumpy (nodular), then the problem is within the tendon itself. Self-massage can be performed with one of the many self massage tools such as The Stick, but avoid the back of the heel area. Focus more on the calf muscles and eliminating any trigger points that may be limiting the motion and proper function of the Achilles.

One good test to determine which structure is causing the injury is to move the tendon through a range of motion. Grasp the painful area and move your foot up and down. If the painful area stays in one place, then it's the paratenon; if the painful area moves, then it's the tendon. Tendinosis responds well to massage directly on the area, whereas paratenodosis responds better to massage above the injured area, up towards the calf muscles.

Strengthening the Achilles

When an Achilles injury starts to enter the chronic stage, which can be as short as two to three weeks after the onset, strengthening exercises need to be added as part of the treatment plan. Start with toe raises of both feet. Build up to 15, and then progress to two sets, using pain and fatigue as your guide. When the exercise becomes difficult or if pain increases, stop at that point.

The next phase is to perform these exercises while isolating the injured limb. Rise up with both feet, and then lift the uninjured foot in the air and drop down slowly on the injured foot. This is known as an eccentric exercise, in which the muscle is lengthening and firing at the same time. Its efficacy for Achilles problems became well-known in 1998, when Dr. Håkan Alfredson published a study on treating chronic Achilles tendinosis. Thirty recreational runners were split into two equal groups. The group that was rehabbed using eccentric exercises all returned to running in twelve weeks. The group that was rehabbed using only rest, stretching, orthotic devices, and physical therapy all failed to improve; some were even treated with surgery. Alfredson recommended three sets of 15 repetitions, twice a day, daily, with no off days.

Alfredson reported a 100 percent success rate that has never been replicated in any studies since his paper was published, but there's no doubt that eccentric strengthening combined with other treatments is invaluable in rehabilitating injured tendons. Alfredson's protocol called for the eccentric exercise to be performed on a step, with the goal on the side that is eccentrically firing to drop the heel below the level of the step. I don't recommend dropping below the level of the step, as this can lead to an

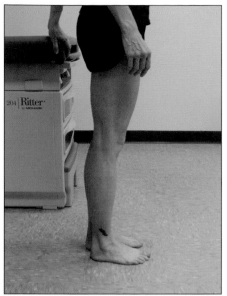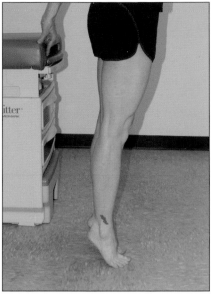

Start with heel raises with both feet. Raise up off both heels, hold for 2-3 seconds and slowly lower back down.

Start with one set and slowly build up to two sets.

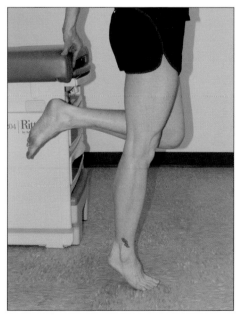

Progress to a one-leg eccentric exercise. Rise up with both feet, lift one foot in the air, and slowly lower down. Build up to two sets of 15 on each leg.

injury of the peroneal tendons or other areas of the back of the foot and heel. The same benefit has been seen in new studies without having the drop go below the level of a step.

It's very important to look above the foot and see how the core muscles are impacting your biomechanics. Strengthening of the hip abductors is often an integral part of the treatment plan. Weakness of the gluteal muscles leads to your trunk dropping down instead of going forward when you run, which not only places more stress on structures such as the Achilles but might also impede performance. (Core exercises are covered in Chapter 6.)

When to Seek Professional Help for Achilles Issues

When you reach the chronic stage, which is typically if the injury is present for longer than two to three weeks, then it's time to see a sports medicine professional. If you've had treatment and aren't improving, then an MRI or diagnostic ultrasound might be recommended to inspect the tendon for cysts or a chronic tear. At the same time, finding the cause of the injury is far more important than anything an MRI or diagnostic ultrasound might reveal. A diagnosis is made by using all the information available. Diagnostic imaging is far from 100 percent reliable versus the actual pathology seen in surgery. MRIs have been found to be much more definitive and sensitive, and to correlate better to what's found if surgery is deemed necessary.

If you're a moderate to severe pronator, then a custom orthotic device may help correct one of the causative factors. Working with a sports physical therapist has been critical to the successful treatment of my patients with this injury. If all of the conservative treatments fail and the injured tendon is preventing normal activity, then using a removable walking boot to completely immobilize the tendon could be considered. Remember that this must be followed by a rehabilitation of the muscles because atrophy will occur from immobilization.

Extracorporeal Shock Wave Therapy (ESWT) has also shown to be very effective in treating this injury. It's more known for use in plantar fasciitis but has shown to be successful for insertional tendon injuries. ESWT theoretically promotes the formation of new blood vessels in the treated area to promote healing of the tissue. The downside is that ESWT can be expensive and most insurance companies don't cover this treatment. Radial soundwave, sometimes called EPAT (Electrical Pulsed Activated Therapy), is another form of shockwave treatment. The device sends a sound wave deep into the Achilles to help the tendon heal. Shockwave has been proven to produce new blood vessels in the area. (The medical term for this is "neovascularization.") One study with the device I use in my practice showed a 78 percent success rate in the Achilles treatment of athletes. The full effect may take up to twenty weeks. (See Chapter 9 for more on shockwave therapy.)

I caution against any of the injectable techniques, such as dry needling, prolotherapy, or homeopathic remedies, because the needles can sometimes lead to more damage than good. Also, to date there are no studies that prove platelet rich plasma or any other blood products work better than placebo. (See Chapter 9 for more on these types of treatments.)

Once all conservative treatments have been exhausted, then surgery is a consideration. Athletes need to understand that surgery isn't a quick fix. I recommend a minimum of six months of high-quality conservative therapy before considering surgical management for most problems. If the surgery has a complication, such as an infection, then it can set the athlete back further. The medical literature reveals a complication rate of 7–13 percent for Achilles tendon surgery. This happens in part because some injuries take longer than others to heal, and every patient is different. Some athletes get injured frequently not because they did anything wrong and not because they received poor medical care, but due to their genetic makeup along with a lot of other factors.

Dr. Amol Saxena, a top sports medicine podiatrist in Palo Alto, California, has successfully operated on the Achilles of many Olympians. When asked when it is time for runners to consider surgery, Saxena responds: "When they have done all the non-surgical things, rested completely from running three to six months, when they have pain after every run or they are limping." Overall, 90 percent get better without surgery. The majority of Dr. Saxena's patients get back to prior activity levels within two to six months, depending on the severity of the surgery. (See Chapter 8 for more on surgery for the Achilles.)

Shin Splints

What most people call shin splints is more properly known as medial tibial stress syndrome (MTSS). That term better defines the pain, which occurs along the inside or medial border of the tibia (shin bone). The pain is thought to be due to the attachment of the muscle pulling away from the bone, leading to an inflammation of fascia, which provides an interface between the leg muscles and the tibia. Dr. Rich Bouche, who is one of

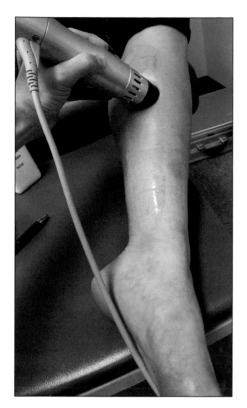

Patient being treated with ESWT for MTSS. The probe is applied to what's known as the posterior medial border. The area shown is the normal range where pain is felt.

the top experts in the country on exercise-induced leg pain, refers to this injury as tibial fasciitis.

There are intrinsic and extrinsic factors causing this injury. These include: gastrocnemius-soleus tightness, deep posterior muscle group weakness, tibial varum (bow legs), improper biomechanics, training on hard surfaces, training errors, and worn-out running shoes. Typically, people with MTSS feel a lot of pain at the start of a run, decreased pain throughout the run, but then increased pain after running. MTSS pain often occurs along the lower third of the posterior medial (back inside) surface of the tibia, which coincides with the origin of the posterior tibial muscle and the soleus muscle. Two different high-level medical studies found that a pronated foot type was statistically significant for predicting MTSS to occur in U.S. Navy recruits and high school runners, respectively.

In chronic cases of MTSS, you'll feel pain with palpation and palpable scar tissue along a diffuse portion of the medial tibia. When you have pain that increases during runs, pain that is more pinpoint with palpation or pain that doesn't resolve with rest and treatment, you should get a bone scan or MRI to check for a possible stress fracture.

Self-treatment should involve icing and stretching. One good way to ice is to freeze small paper cups filled with water. The top of the cup can be peeled away to perform an ice massage of the area. Calf stretching and massage of the calves should also be implemented. Check the wear on your running shoes and consider a new pair of shoes if there are significant signs of wear. Try to run on a softer surface, as impact forces on a harder running surface can lead to more shin pain. Custom orthotic devices can be another effective treatment. ESWT can be a very effective additional treatment, because the fascial border doesn't have a good blood supply. The sound waves can also help to reduce pain, which is a very important aspect of treatment. It's important to note that treatment of MTSS requires addressing multiple areas of the body both above and below the painful area.

Chronic Exertional Compartment Syndrome

If you experience an increase in pain in the calf or front of the leg to the point where you can't finish runs and/or it feels like your foot slaps the ground when you run, you should be checked for chronic exertional compartment syndrome. Another symptom is significant pain at a similar point in each run, which some describe as a feeling of such tightness that it feels as if the calf is about to explode.

John Walker, the 1976 Olympic 1,500-meter champion and the first runner to break 3:50 for the mile, suffered from this injury during his career. He was able to run for 30 minutes before the pain would set in and prevent any further training. Until he had surgery to correct the injury, he would run as hard as he could twice a day for thirty minutes to maximize his training.

The leg is divided into four compartments, each surrounded by fascia, the non-elastic covering that provides the infrastructure of our body. For people suffering from compartment syndrome, the muscles will swell and begin to compress the nerve, causing severe pain that subsides when you stop running. The injury typically only happens during running, so people with it can cross-train pain-free.

Surgery has been found to be the only cure for this injury. Olympians Dick Quax, Mary Slaney, and John Walker all had successful surgery for it and continued their running careers. The surgery involves cutting and releasing the entire length of the fascia within the affected compartment. Most commonly the front of the leg, or anterior compartment, is affected and leads to the foot slapping the ground during a run, as the nerve in that compartment supplies the muscles that dorsiflex or pull the foot up towards the leg. The deep posterior compartment is the second most common compartment effected; pain in that area can more closely mimic medial tibial stress syndrome previous.

Diagnosis is made by measuring the pressures within the compartments with a small device that has a needle attached. This needle is inserted into each compartment. Pressure measurements are typically done prior to exercise. The patient then runs until the symptoms occur. The pressures are measured immediately after and five minutes later, and if the number is elevated, then a diagnosis of compartment syndrome can be made. Normal pressures should be <15 mm Hg at rest, < 30 mm Hg one minute after running, and < 20 mm Hg five min-utes after running.

The Posterior Tibial Tendon

The posterior tibial tendon runs behind the ankle and attaches to the inside of the foot onto the navicular bone. The tendon helps support the arch, and is activated several times during the gait cycle to help decelerate the foot after foot strike. It also helps to re-supinate the foot to prepare for propulsion or toe-off.

You'll feel pain in a similar location to the Achilles as the tendon runs behind the medial malleolus (inside ankle bone). There are four stages of this injury. The initial stage involves tendinitis and pain that can be treated with icing, taping, and cutting back on training. It's imperative to not allow the ten-

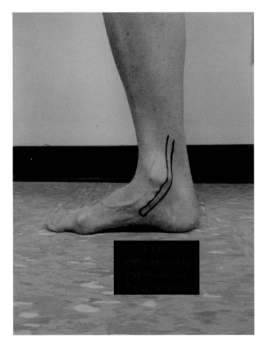

don pathology to progress much past the initial stage. If swelling is seen in the tendon along the inside of the ankle, you must seek medical treatment. The second stage leads to tearing of the tendon and the arch beginning to fall, at which point raising up off the heel on one foot

The medial leg with posterior tibial tendon depicted.

becomes difficult or impossible. Stage 3 advances to more permanent changes of the joints and loss of motion in the joints. Stage 4 is significant pathology with collapse of the tendon and degenerative changes of the joints.

Initially you might feel pain when you rise up on your toes or walk down stairs. As the tendinosis progresses and the tendon degenerates further, there may be tearing in the tendon, which leads to elongation of the tendon and flattening of the arch. If the tendon stretches too much, it will rupture and the arch will collapse. At this stage, surgery is the only solution to correct the problem, and a return to the previous level of function isn't possible.

Another sign of posterior tibial tendon dysfunction is called the "too-many-toes" sign, indicating that if you observe someone barefoot from behind normally you will not see the third, fourth or fifth toes. When you can see three or more toes, it may indicate posterior tibial tendon dysfunction. In advanced stages, the foot will turn out more due to the loss of function of the tendon and collapse of the arch.

Ice and rest are two important aspects of the treatment plan along with extra support in the form of arch supports, good supportive shoes during the day and, sometimes, an ankle brace. There are several well-made lace-up ankle braces that help support the arch and take the pressure off the tendon. Kinesio tape can be used in addition to bracing. Formal physical therapy is a good idea for this injury.

Once the swelling and pain is mitigated then the treatment can move on to strengthening. Strengthening should be performed not just in the foot but also in the core as with most injuries in the foot what happens above the foot can have a major influence on the function of the foot. Start with

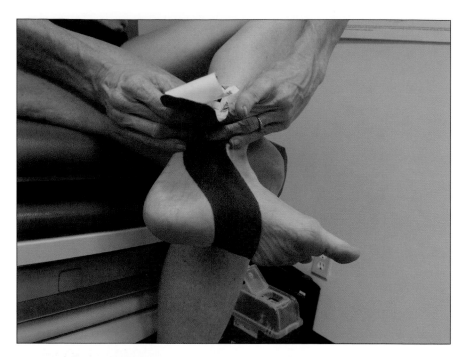

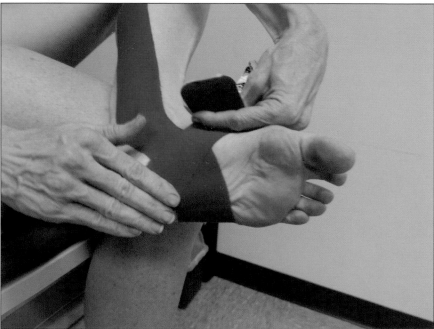

Taping with kinesio tape for posterior tibial tendinosis. Start at the inside of the arch where the tendon inserts. Apply the first 1" without any tension, then put the tape under about a 50 percent stretch (pull to max stretch and back off to get to 50 percent) while applying, following the course of the posterior tibial tendon up the inside of the leg. Place a second strip perpendicular to the portion of the tendon where it's painful.

theraband exercises, progress to heel raises with both feet and eventually to eccentric heel raises on one foot. These exercises and core strengthening exercises such as planks and bridge-ups are covered in detail in Chapter 6.

An overly flat foot may require a custom orthotic device. An over-the-counter device may be used initially but for some feet a custom device might be a better choice. The device can have extra posting and support to take the stress off the posterior tibial tendon. A custom ankle foot orthotic (AFO) device can also be fabricated to allow the tendon to heal. In advanced cases, when the tendon has ruptured, the brace can enable carrying out activities of daily living.

Shockwave therapy is an excellent choice, as it leads to angiogenesis, which is the formation of new blood vessels in the area of the treatment. This process helps the tendon heal better because tendons are poorly vascularized (i.e., they don't receive much blood flow).

Surgery isn't a very good option for a runner, but if the tendon has progressed to Stage 3 or Stage 4, then adaptive changes will occur in the foot, requiring surgical management to be able to function. Surgery will not only repair the ruptured tendon but also require fusions of several of the joints along the medial or inside of the foot. The procedure will lead to compensatory changes in other joints and difficulty running. So again, don't let things get to that stage.

The Peroneal Tendons

The peroneus longus and peroneus brevis tendons are on the outside or lateral aspect of the leg. The two muscles originate next to each other in the lower leg and become tendons as they

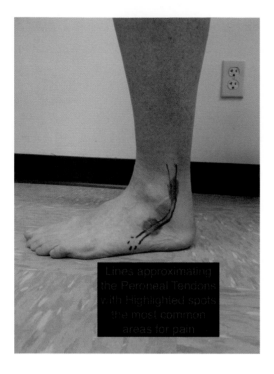

The lateral aspect of leg with the most common painful areas of the peroneal tendons highlighted.

course down towards the foot and travel behind the lateral malleolus (ankle bone). The peroneus brevis attaches to the base of the fifth metatarsal. The peroneus longus dives under the outside of the foot, running under the cuboid in the peroneal groove to attach to the bottom of the base of the first metatarsal. These two tendons serve to decelerate the foot at foot strike and evert (turn out) the foot. The longus tendon also helps to stabilize the first metatarsal by pulling down on it to prepare the foot for toe-off.

The peroneals can be injured from an ankle sprain. They can also develop a tear within the substance of the tendon from overuse or if the tendon doesn't stay in place when it courses behind the lateral malleolus (ankle bone). If a click is felt behind the ankle, then the ligaments that hold the peroneal tendons in place as it goes into the foot could be torn. The tendons run within a groove behind the back of the fibula bone. If the groove isn't deep enough, that can lead to subluxation, in which the tendons dislocate from behind the fibula. This leads to fraying and, eventually, tearing of the tendons.

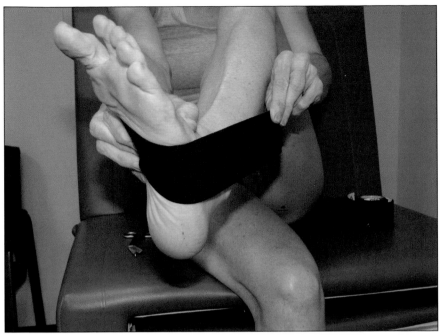

Kinesio taping for peroneal tendon injury. Start under the foot with first 1"
under no stretch, then apply a 50 percent stretch and apply to the skin along
the course of the tendon.

A more neutral shoe and removal of any pronation-
controlling inserts can help peroneal tendinosis improve. The
goal is to offload the lateral aspect
of the leg. Felt can be applied to
the bottom of the sock liner of the
running shoe on the lateral aspect
to tilt the foot towards the midline
of the body. Taping and icing are
also very effective.

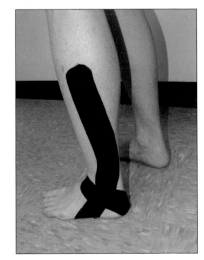

Second strip of tape applied over the
most painful area. Apply tension over the
tendon and lay the tape on each side with
no tension.

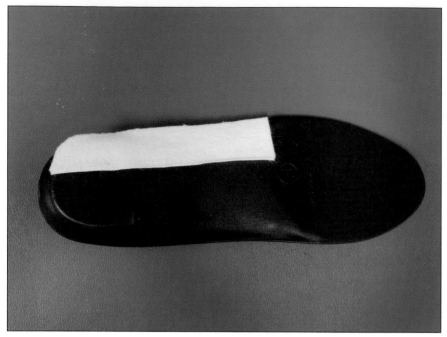

Felt modification for lateral ankle and peroneal pain. Apply 1/8" adhesive felt to the bottom of a sock liner.

Surgery may need to be considered in cases resistant to conservative treatment or if there is a significant tear of the tendons. (See Chapter 8.)

Flexor Hallucis Longus Tendinosis

The flexor hallucis longus (FHL) tendon can develop tendinosis in two main locations: in the arch and behind the ankle. The FHL tendon helps to support the arch and also pulls the hallux (big toe) down towards the ground. The tendon runs behind the ankle, traveling behind a groove in the talus bone, and can become impinged in that area, causing pain and sometimes tearing of the tendon. (It's a common injury in ballet dancers, as the extreme pointing down of the foot at the ankle can pinch the

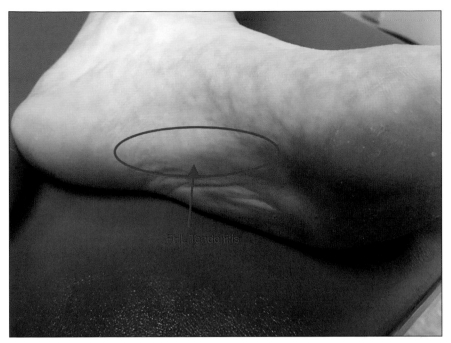

Foot with swelling around the flexor hallucis longus tendon showing where this tendinosis will occur in the arch; not to be confused with plantar fasciitis.

tendon.) The back of the talus bone is known as the posterior talar process, which sometimes is larger than normal or even may be a separate bone, in which case it's called an os trigonum.

Due to the close proximity to the Achilles tendon, FHL pathology in back of the talus can be mistakenly thought to be Achilles tendinopathy. Tendinopathy in this area responds well to a cortisone injection, but it's important to determine if there's a problem with the bone, and whether there's a fracture of the posterior process or just inflammation from an enlarged bone. In some instances, surgical removal of the os trigonum may be necessary. For an injection, it's best to approach the tendon from the lateral side of the foot to avoid damage to the nerve that runs on the medial or inside of the ankle bone.

When the pain is located in the arch of the foot, it can sometimes have an associated swelling. The treatment in the arch is very similar to plantar fasciitis treatment, responding well to icing, taping, and arch support. Taping is similar to plantar fascia taping. ESWT will be very effective for this injury as well. Surgery should ideally be avoided when the injury location is in the arch of the foot, due to the many layers of muscles and the plantar fascia that need to be cut through to reach the FHL tendon.

Final Thought

An injured tendon can develop into a more chronic and difficult injury than most other injuries, including fractures. If swelling is noted and at-home remedies of ice and rest don't help enough, then seek treatment from your local sports podiatrist. As with most injuries, the sooner it is treated, the faster you can return to running.

Chapter Five
Stress Fractures

Treating stress fractures in athletes can be challenging. Runners who participate in school, professionally, or at the highest local levels often have a narrow time frame to train and compete in their desired sporting activities. Reducing healing time by every means possible is crucial to the success of these athletes. For some, running is their main form of exercise and stress relief, so returning to training can be just as important to the recreational runner. The goal of any sports medicine professional should always be to return the athlete back to activity as soon as is safely possible for the athlete.

Stress fractures were first described in 1855 as "march fractures" by the Prussian military surgeon Breithaupt, who made the clinical description of swelling and pain in feet with a metatarsal stress fracture. The fractures were closely associated with the marching done by soldiers. In 1897, with the advent of X-rays, it was possible to see stress fractures in military recruits forced to go on long marches, thereby establishing the association between stress fractures and overuse. In modern times, many competitive athletes will straddle the fine line between optimal fitness and injury to achieve the best performance possible, making them susceptible to this injury.

In 1987, a landmark paper by Dr. Gordon Matheson, the former chief of sports medicine at Stanford University, analyzed stress fractures (as verified via bone scans) in 320 athletes from a variety of sports, of which 221 were runners with an average weekly mileage between twenty-seven and forty-four miles. He assessed the results of conservative management. The most common bone injured was the tibia (49.1 percent), followed by the tarsals (25.3 percent), metatarsals (8.8 percent), femur (7.2 percent), fibula (6.6 percent), pelvis (1.6 percent), sesamoids (0.9 percent), and spine (0.6 percent). Stress fractures were on both sides (bilateral) in 16.6 percent of cases.

When to Suspect a Stress Fracture

The most common site of a stress fracture in the lower body is the tibia (shin bone), followed by the metatarsals, the bones in the foot behind the toes. Most stress fractures develop gradually. The pain may initially be noticed after a hard training session or race, or the morning after a long or difficult workout.

Typically, the pain will become more focused in a small area as the fracture develops. Localized swelling might be noticed in the area as well. The pain will get worse during a run and may become sharp enough to force you to end the run. The pain will linger after the run is over and might still be felt when you're not on your feet after activity. While not the case for every injury, a soft-tissue injury such as tendonitis will hurt more with your first steps and then perhaps not hurt as much as you warm up. In contrast, a stress fracture hurts more as the activity progresses. If you keep training on a nascent stress fracture, thc pain can become worse as the workout goes on until the fracture becomes more fully developed.

Don't think that your injury is a stress fracture only if you're unable to run. Athletes tend to have high levels of pain tolerance, and while working out, endorphins are released that can further mask the pain. For example, Rich Kenah won bronze medals at 800 meters in the 1997 indoor and outdoor world

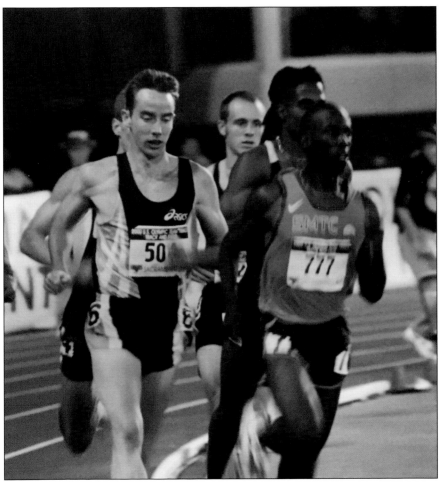

Rich Kenah (#50) competing in the 2000 U.S. Olympic Trials. Rich overcame two stress fractures in the preceding years to make the Olympics in the 800 meters.

championships. Early in his build-up for the 1998 season, Rich began experiencing pain in the middle of his foot; it was eventually diagnosed as a navicular stress fracture. Rich was able to continue to train despite the stress fracture, and in the process of compensating for the pain he developed a second stress fracture in the fourth metatarsal of the same foot. Fortunately, Rich eventually healed both fractures and made the U.S. Olympic team in 2000.

Causes of Stress Fractures

Much of the literature points to overuse as one of the main causes of a stress fracture. Overuse or training errors can account for the extrinsic factors in an injury, but intrinsic factors such as poor bone density, low body weight, low vitamin D levels, weakness of the core musculature, and biomechanical abnormalities, including limb-length differences, can all lead to a stress fracture.

A Stanford University study by Dr. Michael Fredericson found that athletes who played ball sports such as basketball or soccer during childhood had a decreased incidence of stress fractures as adults. A correlation can be made that these athletes developed better core musculature, in particular the hip abductors, leading to fewer injuries. Athletes are often searching for ways to improve performance. Adding a core-strengthening program is arguably the best way to help prevent injury leading to improved performance. We'll look at core strength in detail in the following chapter.

Injured athletes should always be questioned about their dietary habits, in particular their intake of dietary calcium and vitamin D. A Stanford study from 2010 showed a decrease in stress fractures in runners when there was an increase in their dietary calcium and vitamin D intake. Our bodies will typically absorb roughly half of the listed amount of a supplement, so keep that in mind if sun exposure isn't practical or possible. Also keep in mind that our body absorbs vitamins better from food sources—in this case, primarily dairy products—than supplements.

A referral to an endocrinologist is appropriate when an athlete presents with multiple stress fractures in a short time. It's imperative to check the blood levels of vitamin D for any runner with a stress fracture. The blood test checks serum 25-hydroxy-vitamin D (25(OH)D). Many labs will list a "normal" range of 30-70 ng/ml, but 30 may be too low for an athlete. Low vitamin D levels lead to increased bone turnover, which increases the risk for a bone injury like a stress fracture. A study examining male Finnish military recruits found vitamin D status to be a significant determinant of maximal peak bone mass and also discovered that levels below 30 ng/mL significantly increased the risk of stress fractures in this subject group. Many experts recommend a minimum level of 75-90 nm/ml for athletes.

The sun is the best source of vitamin D. Less than fifteen minutes of exposure per day can help to provide the proper daily dosage. The prevention of skin cancer dictates the use of sunscreen, but an SPF of 15 will block 99 percent of the body's production of this natural source of vitamin D.

In November 2010, the Institute of Medicine released new recommendations for dietary intake of vitamin D: 400–600 IU/day for children and adults (0–70 years), 800 IU/day for older adults (>70 years). These values are only slightly higher than past recommendations and are too low for athletes. The Endocrine Society recommends 400–1000 IU/day for infants,

600–1000 IU/day in children (1–18 years) and 1500–2000 IU/day in adults, in addition to sensible sun exposure.

Based on research presented on recovery, force, and power production, 4000–5000 IU/day of vitamin D3 in conjunction with a mixture of 50 mcg/day to 1000 mcg/day of vitamin K1 and K2, seems to be a safe dose and has the potential to aid athletic performance. Make sure to use this dose of vitamin D only if your levels have been checked and noted to be low. Blood levels of vitamin D need to be monitored if you are supplementing at this level because it's a fat-soluble vitamin and toxicity can occur if the levels become too high. The main consequence of vitamin D over dosage is hypercalcemia, a build-up of calcium in your blood that can lead to a decreased appetite, weakness, nausea, and, in severe cases, kidney problems.

Women can have a harder time maintaining and improving bone health. The older terminology that addressed female athletes and bone health was known as Female Athlete Triad Syndrome. Relative Energy Deficiency in Sport (RED-S) is the new term, which includes male athletes as well. For women, the three components of the triad were amenorrhea, anorexia, and osteoporosis. We have come to understand that this issue is much more complex. An editorial in the *British Journal of Sports Medicine* summarized the terminology change and the reasons for it:

> The syndrome of RED-S refers to impaired physiological function including, but not limited to, metabolic rate, menstrual function, bone health, immunity, protein synthesis, cardiovascular health caused by relative energy deficiency. The cause of this syndrome is energy deficiency relative to the balance between dietary energy

intake and energy expenditure required for health and activities of daily living, growth and sporting activities. Psychological consequences can either precede RED-S or be the result of RED-S. The clinical phenomenon is not a 'triad' of the three entities of energy availability, menstrual function and bone health, but rather a syndrome that affects many aspects of physiological function, health, and athletic performance. This Consensus Statement also recommends practical clinical models for the management of affected athletes. The 'Sport Risk Assessment and Return to Play Model' categorizes the syndrome into three groups and translates these classifications into clinical recommendations.

Diagnosis of Stress Fractures

If you have pain of the sort described above that gets worse as your run progresses, then a visit to the podiatrist should be the next step. Remember, stress fractures are often the opposite of soft-tissue injuries, which typically hurt more at the start of a run.

Successful conservative treatment of a stress fracture is extremely dependent on the timely diagnosis and initiation of treatment. Palpation of the injured area and careful documentation of the injury history are key components of making a proper diagnosis. One diagnostic test that works well is having the patient hop on the injured side. This may produce sharp, pinpoint pain if a fracture is present. One may also use the hop test to help determine if the bone is healed enough to return to activity.

Most physicians have radiographs readily available. With the advent of digital X-ray equipment, it's possible to pick up a stress fracture earlier than ever. It's important to keep in mind that negative radiographs should almost never rule out a stress fracture. I've treated patients with a stress fracture diagnosed via an MRI and/or bone scan where the fracture never revealed itself in a plain radiograph. In the following two images, the patient had pain and swelling but no signs of a fracture in the

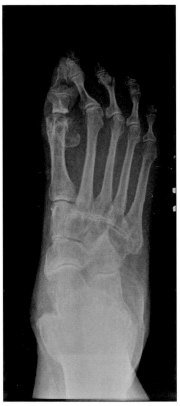 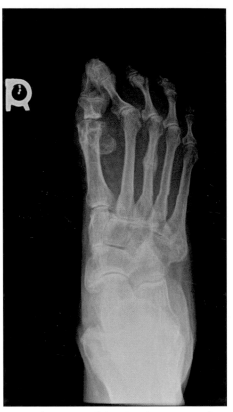

Note almost no change in third metatarsal. Patient had pain and swelling in foot.

Stress fracture of the third metatarsal clearly evident. Note the prior surgery on the big toe joint leading to more stress on the other metatarsals. At the time of the X-ray most of the pain and swelling is gone. It's important not to use the results of an X-ray or other test as the only determining factor in regards to healing.

first X-ray. While the second X-ray of the same patient four weeks later shows the fracture, by this point most of the patient's pain had disappeared.

Some bones, such as the navicular or cuboid, may never exhibit radiographic changes in the presence of a stress fracture. While metatarsal stress fractures can sometimes be seen on X-ray, it's sometimes not until symptoms have subsided that there's radiographic evidence of bone healing.

If initial radiographs are negative and further testing is required, then the physician can choose among diagnostic ultrasound, MRI, bone scan, CT scanning, or some combination. There's some debate as to whether MRI or bone scan are better for diagnosing a stress fracture. One study showed that a bone scan is much more sensitive, whereas MRI can be more specific for detecting the exact location for the injury.

One must use caution in interpreting MRI results as bone marrow edema, which is commonly associated with a stress reaction or stress fracture, can also be seen in asymptomatic individuals. A colleague once had a patient who was being evaluated for a sesamoid injury via MRI of the feet and legs as a screening prior to signing a professional soccer contract.

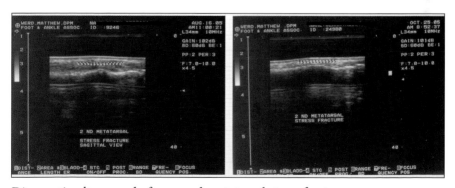

Diagnostic ultrasound of a second metatarsal stress fracture.
Image courtesy of Dr. Matt Werd.

The athlete had spent the morning practicing with a lot of ball strikes, and the MRI was read as multiple stress fractures of the metatarsals despite the fact that the patient had no symptoms in that area. Some doctors have diagnostic ultrasound available in their office. It can be a great way to evaluate soft tissue pathology and can also detect a stress fracture much earlier than a regular X-ray. The value of readings from the units are very much dependent on the expertise of the user.

A CT scan is a much better option for some bones, such as the navicular or cuboid, and when an MRI is inconclusive and shows an increase of bone marrow edema. Computerized tomography visualizes the cortex of bone much better than MRI.

A variant of the CT scan is the SPECT-CT, which combines nuclear medicine similar to a bone scan with a CT scan. SPECT images are obtained following an injection of a radiopharmaceutical that's used for bone scans. The injected medication travels to areas where the bone is fractured and will highlight the injured area. The radiopharmaceutical is detected by a gamma camera. The camera or cameras rotate over a 360-degree arc around the

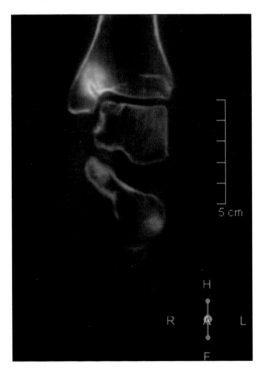

Stress fracture of the medial ankle bone revealed on SPECT-CT.

Image courtesy of Dr. Amol Saxena.

patient, allowing for reconstruction of an image in three dimensions.

General Treatment of Stress Fractures

Stress fractures are one of the few athletic injuries that can require an almost complete cessation of weight-bearing exercise. A good general rule of thumb to guide treatment is that anything that causes pain should be avoided. One exception to this rule has been created with the AlterG treadmill, which creates a vacuum around the runner and allows running at a reduced body weight. (More on this technology in Chapter 9.)

Bone healing of a fracture generally takes four to six weeks, but there are many factors that influence that time frame. The

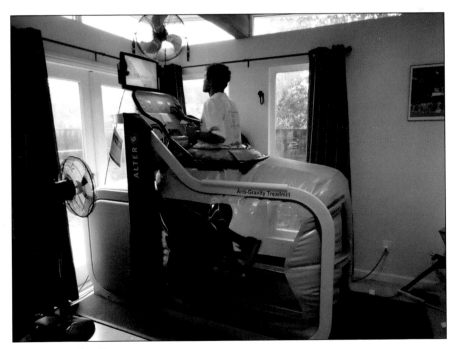

AlterG treadmill.
Photo courtesy of Dr. Amol Saxena

most important factor is which bone is injured and the location within the bone. For example, a stress fracture in the middle of the second, third and fourth metatarsals can heal and allow a return to running within four weeks. In contrast, a navicular stress fracture requires up to eight weeks of non-weight bearing in a cast, and on average takes at least three months to return to full training. While you're waiting for a stress fracture to heal, make sure your diet includes a good amount of foods high in calcium and vitamin D.

Return to running is based on the complete absence of pain when pressing on the fracture spot as well as being able to hop on one foot. Run on softer surfaces such as grass if possible and include one to two days off after each run for the first couple of weeks. You might notice some aching in the site of the stress fracture and occasionally pain after a run, which can linger for months after the fracture heals. Be sure to back off if pain increases during a run or if the pain feels similar to the original pain of the stress fracture. My golden rule: if you have a limp when you run, then you shouldn't be running, as you may end up with a different injury due to compensation.

Extracorporeal Shock Wave Therapy (ESWT) shows promise in reducing healing times for stress fractures. One study examined five athletes who had delayed or non-unions of stress fractures. Once treated with ESWT, each injury showed significant improvements, leading the study authors to opine that ESWT promotes the formation of new bone and helped these athletes heal faster. ESWT is a noninvasive and effective treatment for resistant stress fractures. Similar to the use of bone stimulation, there are no known negative effects for the use of shock wave therapy for stress fractures. Let's look in detail at the most common sites of stress fractures in runners.

Metatarsal Stress Fractures

If you have pain on the top of the foot accompanied by swelling, suspect a metatarsal stress fracture. The pain can range from an ache when the fracture is first developing to sharp shooting pain. You'll usually feel more pain at toe-off. Compare the injured foot to the uninjured foot. If you pull your toes up away from the ground, you'll normally see the five extensor tendons that help to move the toes up pretty clearly. But in the case of a stress fracture the swelling in the area of the fracture will obscure the ability to see these tendons.

Two simple tests at home to help figure out if you have a stress fracture are to press over the area and find a spot that causes sharp pain and to hop on one foot for a minute. If the pain increases while you're hopping or if the pain is so sig-

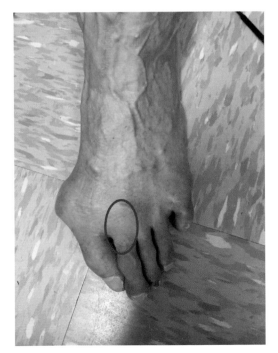

nificant that you have to stop immediately, you may have a stress fracture.

A visit to the sports podiatrist will usually start with a plain X-ray.

Note the subtle difference in swelling behind the second toe in the foot on the right. This would be difficult to detect without a comparison to the unaffected foot. The patient was found to have a stress fracture of the second metatarsal.

It's very important to understand that the fracture may not show up on an X-ray, which shouldn't be the last test performed if it doesn't indicate a break. Your podiatrist might have a diagnostic ultrasound machine, which is another method that can be used to detect a stress fracture. If the fracture isn't discovered with in-office diagnostic testing, then an MRI, a bone scan, or CT scan may be the next test ordered by your doctor.

These long, thin bones are subject to significant ground reaction forces during running, which can lead to a break in one of the cortices. In a cross-section the bone is square-shaped with four distinct sides. A stress fracture will sometimes not show on radiograph until it's healing because it's not completely through the bone and may involve only one of the four sides.

The length pattern of the bones can predispose a bone that is longer than the first metatarsal to extra stress. Pain will be felt most at toe-off and/or impact.

Use of a surgical shoe (a stiff-soled shoe also known as a fracture shoe) to offload the painful area will often suffice for metatarsal stress fractures. If you have pain when walking in a surgical shoe, then it may be necessary to move to a CAM walker, a removable, short leg cast boot. If pain is still noted then non-weight bearing may be warranted.

The location of the fracture is another important consideration. If the fracture is farther away from the toes than the halfway point of the bone, then no weight bearing might be required. A medical scooter, which allows the injured leg to rest on the scooter, can make it much easier to get around compared to crutches.

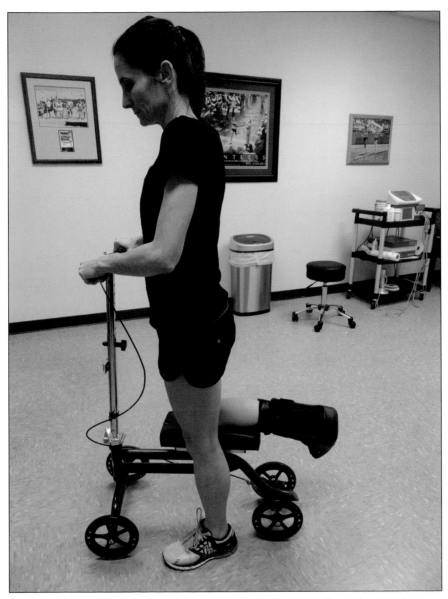

A medical scooter allows much more mobility than crutches when you're keeping weight off an injured foot.

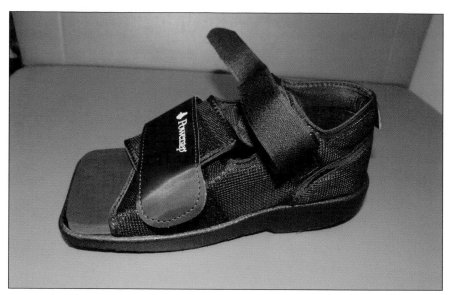

Surgical or fracture shoe, a stiff-soled shoe that doesn't bend, allowing forefoot injuries to heal better.

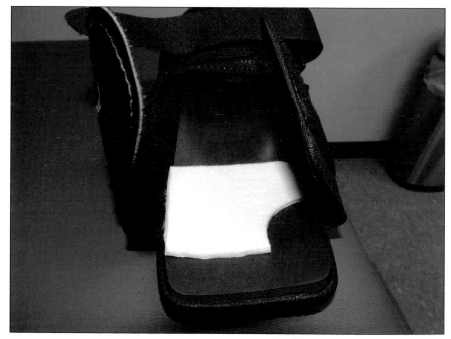

Surgical shoe with 1/8" adhesive felt cutout to help take more pressure off the painful area, in this case for pain in the ball of the foot under the big toe joint.

Navicular Stress Fractures

Navicular stress fractures have been found to occur in runners at a surprisingly high rate and require more aggressive initial treatment than most other stress fractures. A stress fracture of this bone requires complete non-weight bearing, use of a CAM walker, and no exercises that involve movement of the foot, including swimming or other cross training methods that are usually acceptable for a stress fracture of a different bone.

Pain can be non-specific with this injury and may not be felt in one particular spot while running. In classic cases there's pain in the top of the foot when pressing over the navicular, which is called the N spot. Pain may radiate away from this area, but pressing on the N spot can reveal significant pain. A good test at home to stress the area is to crouch down like a baseball catcher. And a second test is to hop up and down on the

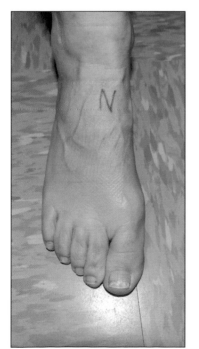

injured foot to assess for pain. The navicular is in the middle of the foot. When viewing the foot from the side the bone is the apex or highest point of the foot. The bone is subject to some unique impact forces owing to the location in the foot and the anatomy of the bones around it.

The Matheson study mentioned earlier in this chapter found that 25 percent of the fractures were of

The N spot, the area where a navicular stress fracture will hurt with a fracture.

tarsal bones, which includes the navicular. The diagnosis and treatment of navicular stress fractures can be difficult, because the symptoms don't always occur right over the bone and initial X-rays will rarely reveal signs of a fracture. The gold standard of conservative treatment consists of eight to ten weeks of immobilization, including no weight bearing. This is one of the few injuries where it's best to not do any cross training that involves the foot, even pool running, because the tendons that insert around the bone can stress the area and delay healing.

I co-authored a paper with Dr. Amol Saxena and Dr. Dave Hannaford that proposed a classification system for the treatment of these injuries based on CT findings that's both prognostic and diagnostic. The classification is divided in to type 1, a fracture through one cortex of the bone; type 2, a fracture that extends into the body of the bone; and type 3, a complete fracture. We found in our studies that type 1 responds best to conservative treatment and type 3 responds best to surgical treatment, consisting of a screw to stabilize and help the fracture site heal. The injury will take an average of three to four months to return to activity. There may be an associated degenerative change in the talo-navicular joint that can cause pain years after a navicular stress fracture.

Making an early and accurate diagnosis is paramount to successful treatment and to lessen the chance of future arthritic-type changes. An initial radiograph may sometimes reveal the fracture but that generally means it could be a complete fracture. If I suspect a navicular stress fracture, my next test after a radiograph is often a bone scan. If the bone scan is negative then you do not have a bone injury or stress fracture. A positive bone scan can be followed up with a CT scan, which will assess the severity of the fracture.

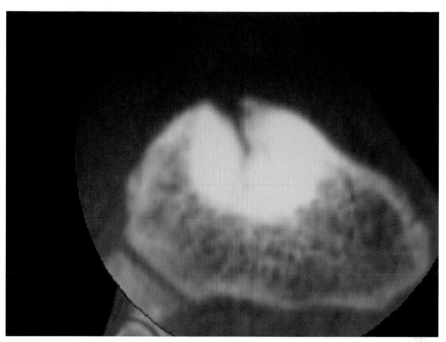

CT scan of the same navicular clearly showing the fracture. A CT scan can better identify a bone injury, especially for the navicular bone.

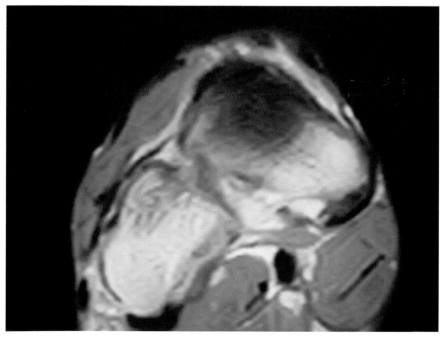

MRI of navicular stress fracture, read as "no fracture" by a radiologist.

Many physicians will automatically order an MRI as the next diagnostic study after an X-ray. Doing so could lead to missing some fractures, as the MRI exam isn't as good as a CT scan for evaluating an older fracture. The two prior photos are an MRI and a CT scan of the same foot a week apart; both were read as "no fracture" by the radiologist. (In fairness to radiologists, they usually don't have the benefit of physically examining the patient.) The CT scan clearly shows the fracture while the MRI showed bone marrow edema, which is sometimes a sign of a fracture.

Calcaneal Stress Fractures

The calcaneus is the main heel bone in the body. It's a dense, thick bone and not a very common spot for a stress fracture, although I have treated as many as three patients in a short time for one. Physicians often initially treat all heel pain as plantar

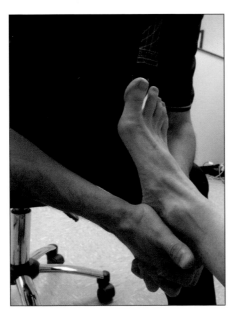

fasciitis, because that's the most common cause of heel pain. Plantar fasciitis usually hurts more with your first steps in the morning and after sitting. A calcaneal stress fracture will hurt more with increased activity and is often lacking that sharp pain with your first steps. The pain may

Squeeze test to check for a possible calcaneal stress fracture.

be noted in a similar location as plantar fasciitis, so try this test: Apply compression on each side of the heel bone in a "squeeze" test of the calcaneus. Grab the heel and interlock your fingers with the hands on either side of the heel and squeeze. If there's pain, you might have a stress fracture.

If pain persists even after taking one to two weeks off from running, and if the pain increases with more activity and time on your feet, then consider a visit to the podiatrist. This isn't an injury to try to train through, because if the fracture line becomes bigger there's a greater potential for non-healing or a complete break, which would require surgery to allow proper healing.

The diagnosis is best confirmed with a bone scan and will rarely show up on an X-ray or diagnostic ultrasound unless the fracture is more advanced. If the fracture does show up on a plain radiograph, it is an indication that the fracture is more severe and the fracture will take longer to heal. In some cases, returning to running can take up to six months.

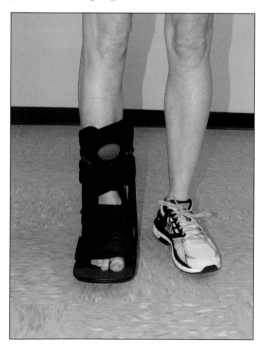

Treatment consists of immobilization in a walking boot and non-weight bearing if walking in the boot is painful. A bone stimulator is a

Short leg walking boot, sometimes called a CAM walker.

good adjunct if possible. Cross training in a pool or other non-impact exercise such as a bike or AlterG are good exercises. If there's pain with any cross training then that exercise should be avoided. If there's pain when swimming with this or any foot injury, put a buoy between your feet and just use your arms.

When I have patients who haven't responded to conservative therapy for plantar fasciitis, I often order another diagnostic test such as an MRI, bone scan, or CT scan. I have found several stress fractures and plantar fascial tears that didn't improve after treatment that usually resolves plantar fasciitis. I suspect that stress fractures of the calcaneus have a great association with lower bone density and low levels of vitamin D as the main causes, as opposed to any biomechanical abnormality.

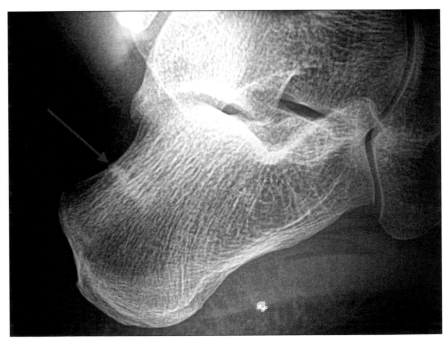

X-ray showing a calcaneal stress fracture in a thirty-year-old woman. She felt sharp pain during a race after having pain for a few weeks.

Sesamoid Stress Fractures

The sesamoid complex consists of two bones under the first metatarsal head (big toe joint). The bones serve to help absorb shock and assist the tendons that pull the hallux (big toe) down (plantar flexion). Owing to a poor blood supply to the area and the small size of the bones, a fracture of these bones often leads to difficulty healing.

Pain will be felt under the ball of the foot. You might feel pain with any motion of the big toe. There may be a feeling of swelling in the area, but it's difficult to see any swelling upon examination. It may sometimes feel as if the big toe joint was jammed or damaged. Any movement of the joint can cause pain due to the fact that the bones are embedded within the tendons that help to move the hallux.

If pain begins in this area, then icing (without placing excess pressure on the area) is important. Avoid high heels, which place much of the body weight directly on the sesamoids. Try to always wear flat, well-cushioned shoes, and avoid barefoot walking if possible. In addition to icing, special pads that can help offload the area are a good first treatment. Dr. Jill's is a company that fabricates a reusable silicone pad called a Dancer's Pad that has a cutout for the sesamoids.

For runners with forefoot pain, I often recommend trying a shoe that has no difference between the height of the heel and the forefoot, or a zero-drop shoe. In a traditional running shoe, the heel is about 12 mm higher than the forefoot. Many companies now offer lower heel heights. Try to find a shoe that has a lower ramp height but is well-cushioned. If switching to a lower-heeled shoe doesn't help to alleviate the pain, then the pain might be caused by more than just inflammation.

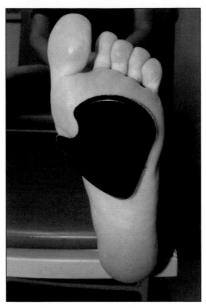

Dr. Jill's Dancer's Pad for sesamoid
pain applied to the foot.

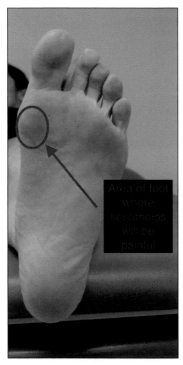

Foot with sesamoids highlighted.

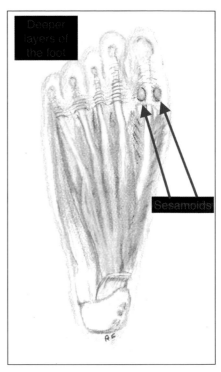

Diagram of sesamoids on bottom of
the foot.

Drawing by Annemarie Fullem, PT.

If pain and swelling persist after resting and attempts to offload the area aren't successful, an X-ray can often detect a stress fracture of the sesamoids. The best treatment is to splint the big toe in a downward (plantarflexed) position and be non-weight bearing for up to six weeks. In less severe cases a surgical shoe with padding to offload the area can work well. Recently, I've been using ESWT on sesamoid injuries with success. The treatment is performed in the office. I typically perform up to five treatments, spaced a week apart. The advantage of the treatment is the production of new blood vessels to the area of the sesamoids, which, as we saw, have a poor blood supply and can be slow to heal.

If the bone does not heal properly and conservative treatment fails, surgery to remove the affected bone may be required.

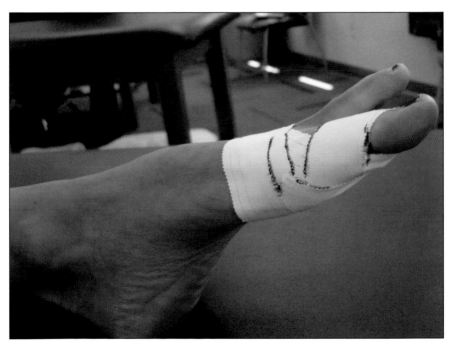

Spica type taping for sesamoid fracture.
Photo courtesy of Dr. Amol Saxena

X-ray of foot from behind highlighting a fractured sesamoid. Note the irregular appearance.

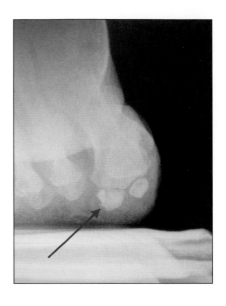

Tim Broe suffered from a fractured sesamoid that failed to heal, and after having the bone removed he won the 2004 U.S. Olympic Trials at 5,000 meters and made the final in the event that year at the Athens Olympic Games. His main event before 2004 was the steeplechase, which may be one of the main reasons he developed a sesamoid fracture. The event features twenty-eight hurdles in less than two miles of running. When hurdling, steeplechasers try to land on the ball of the foot, putting significant stress on the sesamoids.

Tibial Stress Fractures

The tibia (shin) bone can develop stress fractures in several areas. Shin pain along the inside of the leg may initially seem to be "shin splints," which is associated with overuse and stress of the muscles that originate along this bone. (More on this injury in Chapter 4.) The medical term for shin splints is medial tibial stress syndrome (MTSS). Pain from MTSS is usually over a larger area of up to six to eight inches along the front inner shin. Left untreated, the muscles and tendons can create a small crack in the cortex of the bone. The pain from MTSS is worse in the beginning of a run. If pain worsens and

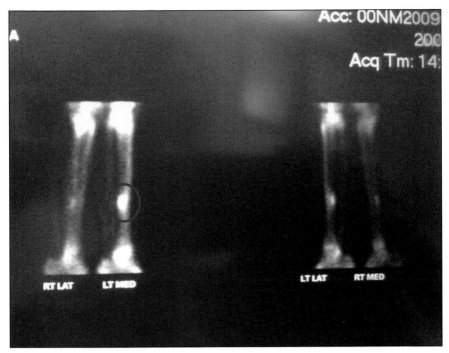

Bone scan revealing a stress fracture of the tibia.

becomes more noticeable over a more discrete area—sometimes the size of a half-dollar coin—then a stress fracture should be suspected.

Self treatment for shin pain should involve increased calf stretching. Hold the stretch for 30 seconds, repeating five times, up to three times per day. The best way to ice this area is with water frozen in a small paper cup; ice along the medial tibial border where the pain is located. Getting on a softer surface and making sure your shoes aren't overly worn are two things I usually recommend to runners with shin pain. Focus on improving your hip abductor strength (see Chapter 6 for core exercises). If you have a flatter foot, an orthotic device can reduce the stress on the muscles attaching the tibia that cause this pain.

Expect the initial X-rays to not reveal the fracture, as these fractures are difficult to detect with radiographs. A bone scan is often the best next diagnostic test to perform.

Treatment typically utilizes a walking boot and possibly being non-weight bearing. With most stress fractures, if there isn't pain while walking in a cast boot or cast shoe, then being non-weight bearing isn't necessary unless the fracture is in an area that has a higher risk of not healing properly such as the navicular, sesamoids, or other area with a poor blood supply.

The most common area in the tibia to develop a stress fracture is in the middle of the bone and along the posterior medial border. This area will usually heal well. But when the fracture is in the front of the tibia (known as the anterior cortex), then the bone may not heal as well since the blood supply to that area of the bone is poor. When an anterior tibial cortex stress fracture is visualized on X-rays this is called the "dreaded black line," which usually indicates that healing has stopped and more drastic measures such as surgery may need to be considered. When the fracture is located in the inside ankle bone that may possibly be easier to detect on X-rays but can be confused with tendonitis, as the posterior tibial tendon courses closely around and under the medial malleolus.

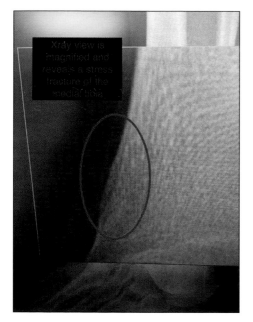

X-ray of stress fracture of a medial malleolus.

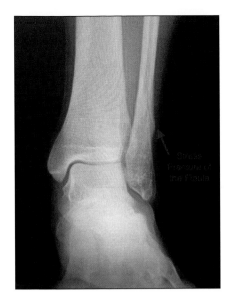

X-ray of fibular stress fracture.

Runners will sustain stress fractures of the other shin bone, the fibula, less often. A higher arch and a supinated foot type can lead to more stress on the lateral aspect of the leg and make the fibula more susceptible to fractures. The good news about the fibula bone is that it doesn't bear as much weight as the tibia, so return to activity can be sooner. Terrell Owens famously played in a Super Bowl with a fibular fracture, but it's certainly not recommended to run if you have pain.

Treatment varies depending on the severity of the fracture and the symptoms, but sometimes just eliminating any impact exercise and cutting back on walking and weight-bearing activity may be enough. A walking cast boot may be needed for a short time until there's no pain with walking.

Chapter Six
Core and Foot Strength

The foot has several muscles that can weaken from being supported in shoes or arch supports. Strengthening these muscles can help the foot and body function better. The muscles in the rest of the leg, especially in the core, have a great impact on the function of the feet. Some injuries of the foot and ankle can improve markedly by improving the functioning of the hip abductors, which for a runner are the most important aspect of the core muscle group. In this chapter we'll look at areas of the body and foot to strengthen to help prevent and resolve injuries as well as improve performance.

The Importance of Core Strength

If I had to choose one group of muscles to strengthen and function better to improve running performance and help prevent injury in the foot and ankle, it would be the core muscles.

Consider: when the foot is in contact with the ground, the body is functioning as a closed chain, which means that everything within that chain has an impact on how the leg functions.

In other words, when the foot is on the ground, the structures and muscles above the foot will affect how the foot is functioning, and vice versa. I've found that a person's back pain can be related to how the foot works, and the foot can be impacted by weakness or imbalances in the muscle groups up to the hip.

One of the most important muscle groups for a runner is the hip abductors, which are located in the outer part of the buttocks. The gluteus medius and gluteus minimus are two of these muscles, and they have a significant effect on foot and leg function. The small muscles and tendons in the feet and legs have a difficult time controlling pronation and resisting the body forces of two to four times your body weight when running. Strong, well-functioning gluteus medius and minimus muscles can help to control motion of the lower extremity and lead to less stress on the foot and ankle structures. For this reason, it's important to assess hip abductor strength and function for most injuries in the lower-extremities.

In 2000, Dr. Michael Fredericson, a sports medicine specialist at Stanford University, discovered that weakness of the hip abductor muscles (mainly the gluteus minimus and gluteus medius) was the leading cause of iliotibial band syndrome. Research since then has shown that Fredericson was correct in his original assumptions. A follow-up study that looked at 3D kinematics of women runners revealed that those who develop iliotibial band syndrome have an increased hip abduction motion, along with greater knee internal rotation, both of which are likely caused by weakness in the hip abductors.

One of my patients highlights the importance of the core muscles to the feet and legs. Ed was a runner in his mid-fifties who hadn't missed a day of running in more than thirty years. During that time he'd run more than thirty consecutive

Boston Marathons. He came to my office in February, about two months before that year's Boston, with a swollen and painful Achilles tendon. This was before the advent of shockwave therapy, which I now use for such injuries. At the time, I often recommended no running if a patient had a swollen Achilles tendon.

Ed told me that he wouldn't consider taking time off, even one day, from running. So we chose to try physical therapy. I referred him to a PT practice that included two runners (one of whom was my wife, Annemarie). Ed was found to have extremely weak hip abductors, which will cause the pelvis to drop and lead to more stress on the lower leg and Achilles tendon. An eccentric strengthening program for the Achilles was instituted along with a core program designed to strengthen the hip abductors. Ed not only kept his running streak intact, but also completed that year's Boston Marathon.

To do the eccentric exercises for Achilles problems, start by performing a heel raise up and down on both feet. Slowly rise up on your toes and hold for a count of two seconds, and then slowly lower the heels down to the ground. When two sets of 15 repetitions can be performed without any increase in pain or difficulty completing them, progress to doing the heel raises one foot at a time.

Here's another example that illustrates the close connection between core strength and healthy feet and ankles. I once had a patient with a diagnosis of posterior tibial tendon dysfunction who hadn't run in eighteen months. During that time she'd had more than twenty sessions of physical therapy. At one point she was placed in a walking cast boot for six weeks. After her pain subsided her sports medicine doctor told her that she could resume running. Unfortunately, she was told this without

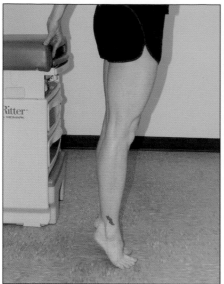 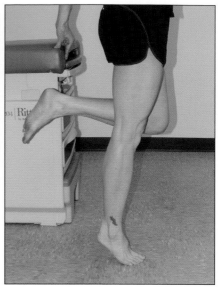

Eccentric Achilles strengthening. Rise up on both feet.

Lift one foot in the air and slowly drop down on the opposite foot. Repeat 15 times on each side and build up to two sets per day.

receiving advice on first correcting the atrophy of muscles that stems from lack of use while in a cast. Her pain returned immediately, and she then went for another course of therapy.

She saw me for another opinion. I didn't see the normal findings associated with this injury; her posterior tibial tendon was very strong. I did, however, note that her hip abductors were extremely weak. I gave her a series of exercises to perform, many of which are detailed in this chapter, and asked her to try to run before returning in a month for a follow-up visit. She was skeptical but on her return visit she was able to run more than a mile pain-free for the first time in almost two years. Her posterior tibial tendon was plenty strong but her core was so weak that her body weight was overwhelming the small tendons in the foot and leg.

A Simple Sample Core Routine

A simple routine of the following exercises can be performed every day. These exercises will improve your core strength and might improve your performance (if for no other reason than you'll be less likely to get injured and can therefore keep training consistently). When doing the exercises, focus on proper form, as described below for each exercise. Maintaining the right form is the most important aspect of all these exercises.

Build to holding each pose for 30 seconds. But again, proper form is paramount. Hold a pose only as long as you can maintain the right form for the exercise. Over time, you'll be able to hold the proper form longer.

Bridge-ups

Lie flat on a table or padded area and bend your knees at close to a right angle with the feet flat on the ground. Raise your

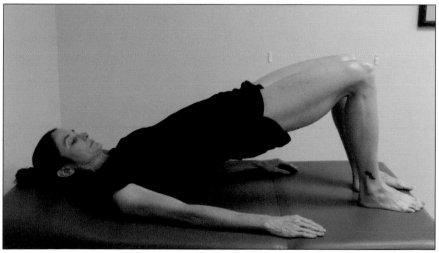

A bridge-up with proper form, showing a straight line from shoulders to knees and pelvis not dropping. Hold for 30 seconds and repeat up to five times as long as you maintain proper form.

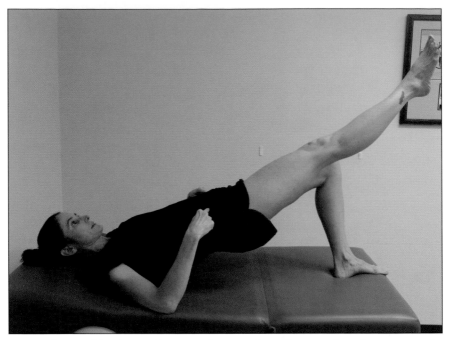

More advanced bridge-up by extending one leg. Alternate legs for 30 seconds and repeat.

trunk up off the table while keeping the feet planted. Aim to form a straight line with your body. The trunk area should stay level and not drop to one side or below the level of the rest of the body.

Hold the pose for 30 seconds or until you notice your body shaking or you have difficulty maintaining proper form.

Planks

Planks are one of the best exercises for any athlete, as they improve the strength of the entire core.

For prone planks (facing down), get into a position similar to how you do a push-up, but resting on your forearms. Bring your whole body off the ground on your toes and try to make a straight line with your body by not allowing your butt to get too high or drop down below the level of the rest of the body. Hold this position for up to 30 seconds.

When the exercise becomes less challenging, you can make it more dynamic by lifting one leg and moving it away from the midline of the body and back. Alternate each leg and build up to five repetitions of each leg while holding the pose for 30 seconds.

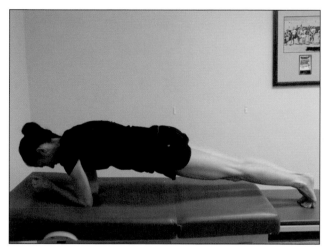

Prone plank with proper form: pelvis is in line with the rest of the body. Hold for 30 seconds if you can maintain your form. Stop with excessive shaking or inability to keep pelvis from dropping.

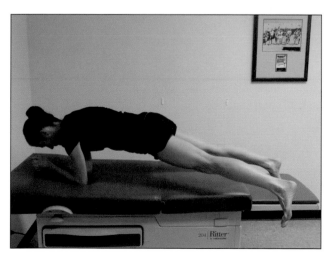

Advanced prone plank: Lifting one leg up and out to side and back to original position. Alternate legs every 2-3 seconds, holding for 30 seconds.

For side planks, prop yourself up on one forearm and the side of one foot. (You might find it easier to keep your shoes on for these.) The key part of the exercise is to form a nice straight line—your pelvis shouldn't drop, or be higher than the rest of your trunk or legs.

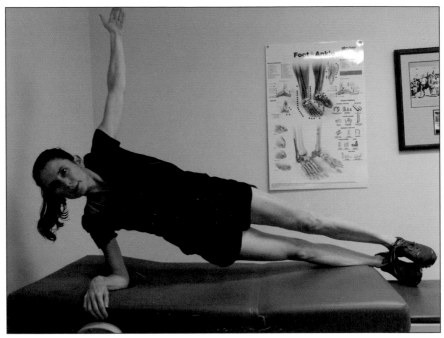

Side plank with proper form; shoulders are perpendicular to the ground with the pelvis staying in line with the rest of the body. Hold for 30 seconds.

If you point the top hand up to the ceiling then your shoulders should be perpendicular to the ground. That's a good indication that you are holding proper form.

When holding the standard side plank position becomes easier, you can add more difficulty by bringing the top leg up in a running motion. Doing so makes the core muscles work even harder to maintain the proper form.

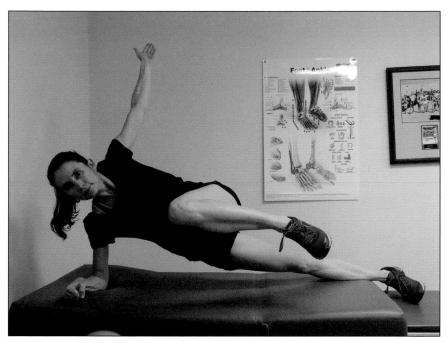

Advanced side plank: bring top leg forward in a running motion for 30 seconds.

¼ Leg Squat

In addition to improving core strength, this exercise can help if you're having knee pain, and it improves your proprioception. Before we describe this particular exercise, let's take a general look at proprioception.

Proprioceptors are sensors in your muscles and tendons that help to govern your balance. Any time you get an injury, these sensors can be damaged. The good news is that if you practice your balance you can repair the proprioceptors, and this will allow your muscles and tendons to function better.

A good way to test your proprioception is to balance on one foot by lifting one foot slightly off the ground and seeing how long you can hold that position without falling to one side. If you can balance without too much trouble, then try the position with your eyes closed. Doing so will cause your body to rely only on your proprioceptors, because your eyes help give feedback to help with balance.

It's fairly typical to find that you're better at balancing on one leg than the other. Make sure to work on both sides to try to get them functioning equally well. If you're not able to balance easily then begin working on your proprioceptors every day by standing on one foot while you brush your teeth and several other times throughout the day. When it becomes easier, balance with your eyes closed until you can hold the position for up to a minute without much difficulty.

For ¼ squats, proper form mainly includes not allowing the knee to drop inside of the foot during the squat. Start by balancing on one foot. Drop down on the standing side so that your knee goes straight over your foot. Drop down about 1/4th of the amount you do in a full squat. Perform the exercise slowly until you no longer can see your toes in front of the knee, and then raise back up. Repeat 15 times per leg for the first 10 days or so. Then

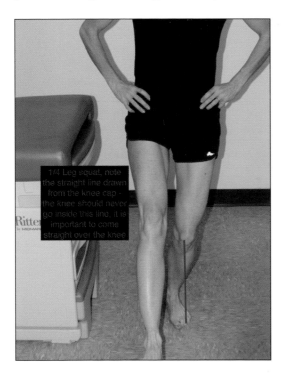

1/4 Leg squat, note the straight line drawn from the knee cap - the knee should never go inside this line, it is important to come straight over the knee

Ritter

¼ leg squat starts by balancing on one foot. Squat down making sure to keep the knee moving straight over the foot; the knee should not go inside of the big toe. Concentrate on keeping the hips level.

begin adding a second set of 15 as tolerated and as long as you're able to maintain proper form. Perform all of these exercises on both legs to avoid muscular imbalances.

Once your balance starts to improve, you can add more movement to the exercises while trying to maintain your balance and proper form. Start with balancing on one foot with the knee slightly bent. Go through a running in place motion with your upper body with a slight forward lean of your body.

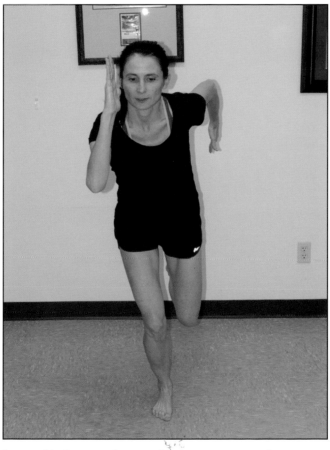

A more advanced balance and strengthening exercise: Balance on one foot with the knee slightly bent. Put your arms through a running motion as if you're running in place with a slight forward lean.

When you're able to complete 30 seconds of this exercise without losing your balance or your form breaking down, the next step is to reach forward to touch the ground.

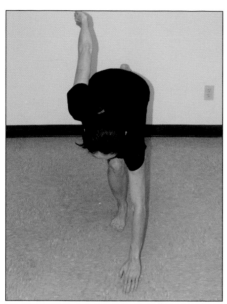

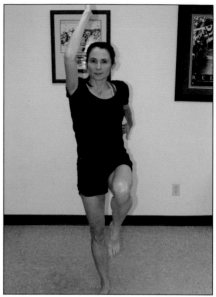

Next level of balance and strengthening: same as last exercise but now reach forward and try to touch the ground.

After touching the ground, reach up to the sky with the same arm.

The next step in this progression adds a soccer ball or basketball to the mix to continue to work the core and proprioceptors. Begin by balancing on one foot with the knee slightly bent. Move the ball from over one shoulder to down below the opposite hip. Keep a chair or stool next to the side and touch the stool with the ball. Try to not allow the knee to move to the inside of your big toe; keep it directly over the foot. Perform the exercise for 30 seconds or until your form breaks down.

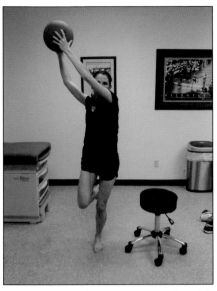
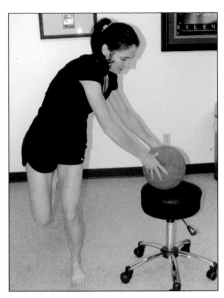

Move the ball from over your shoulder down to the opposite side and touch the stool. Alternate sides.

To make the exercise more challenging, remove the stool and touch the ground with the ball. Start by balancing on one foot with the knee bent. Move the ball from above one shoulder and reach down to the ground on the opposite side of the body.

For a more advanced exercise, add the use of an exercise ball, which will completely isolate your core muscles and not allow recruitment of other muscles to help compensate for weakness in the core group. Start by lying over the ball in

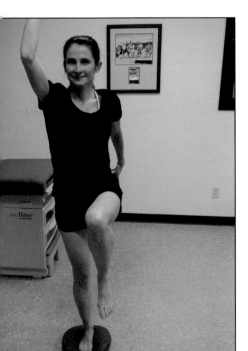

Dynamic proprioception using padding to make the exercise more challenging.

your pelvic area. Spread your legs and keep your feet on the ground. Place your arms on the ground to help balance. You should be able to hold that pose for 30 seconds before moving on the next challenge. Follow the progression as seen in the photos below.

Note that is an advanced exercise and should not be undertaken until you've advanced through a progression of the other exercises.

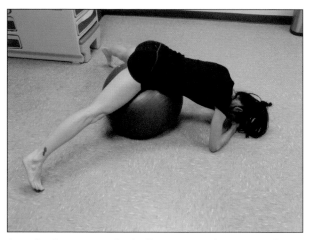

Start by lying over the ball in your pelvic area. This exercise attempts to eliminate recruitment of other muscle groups, keeping the focus on the core.

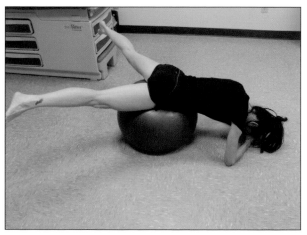

Bring your feet up off the ground.

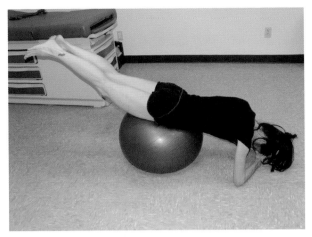

Bring your feet together.

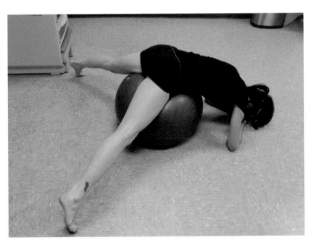

Move feet apart and back down to the ground.

Clamshells

The Thera-Band is a great tool to use to help strengthen many parts of the body. Let's begin with some exercises for the core muscles before moving to strengthening of the foot and ankle.

Clamshells strengthen the gluteal muscles that are so vital to a runner's core. Lie on your side, have your hips bent at a right angle to your torso, and tie a Thera-Band around your legs just above the knees. The tighter the band is around your legs the more resistance it will supply. Open and close your legs slowly, repeating 15 times and building up to two sets on each side.

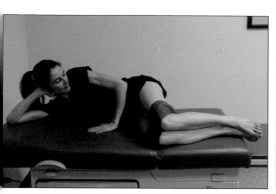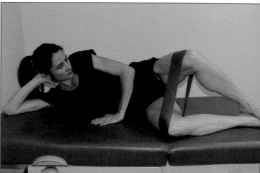

Keep your heels and feet touching each other and open up your legs like a clam shell, imagining that your hips and feet are the hinge to full resistance.

Crab Walks

Another core exercise that uses the Thera-Band for resistance is crab walks. Wrap the band around your knees and crouch

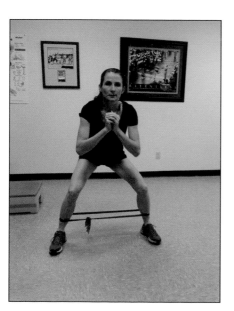

down in a half squat. Stay in the crouched position, move one leg away from the other slowly and move across the room sideways for ten steps.

Crab walks with a Thera-Band: Tie the band below your knees and crouch down by bending your knees. Move your legs sideways, stretching the band to full resistance. Plant the lead foot and bring the legs together. Do 10 steps, then do 10 steps the other direction, leading with the other leg.

Then take 10 steps to return to your starting position while leading with the opposite leg.

Foot and Ankle Strengthening

The Thera-Band is also a great tool to use as the first line of strengthening exercises after an injury such as an ankle sprain or any tendonitis in the foot or ankle. You can wrap one end around the leg of a table to exercise your foot in an inward motion, outward or up towards the front of the leg. You can adjust the amount of resistance by tying the band in a tighter loop or by stretching the band out more before starting the strengthening exercises.

Start with the Thera-Band around the outside of your foot as seen below. Moving your feet to the outside or lateral aspect of your leg will help to strengthen the peroneal muscles. The tendons of these muscles can be damaged in an ankle sprain, or a runner can develop tendonitis from having a higher arched foot that stresses the outside of the foot and ankle too much. Perform two sets of 15, alternating after one set with the exercises described below to create a circuit.

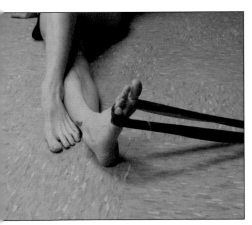 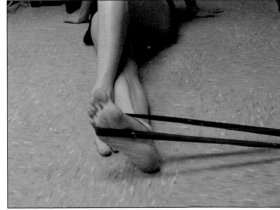

Thera-Band works to strengthen the peroneal muscles.

The second direction is to strengthen the muscles on the inside or medial aspect. Reverse the Thera-Band to be around the foot just behind the big toe joint. Slowly move the foot in an inward-and-up fashion to improve the strength of the posterior tibial tendon and the medial muscles flexor hallucis longus and flexor digitorum longus. Perform two sets of 15 as part of a circuit.

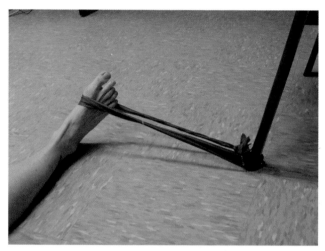

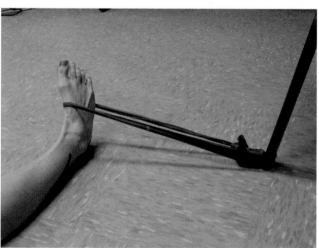

Thera-Band strengthening of the muscles on the medial side, including the posterior tibial muscle.

The third exercise starts with positioning yourself directly in front of the leg of the table, which will allow you to strengthen the anterior muscle group, also known as the dorsiflexors. This muscle group has the muscles that pull the foot up towards the front of the leg. Perform two sets of 15 as part of your circuit.

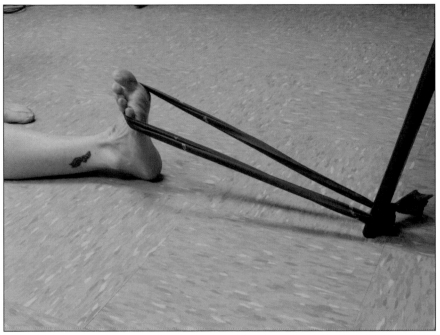

Pull the band up towards the front of your leg slowly. Perform 15 repetitions.

For the fourth direction hold the Thera-Band with each hand and criss-cross over the top of your leg. Apply resistance to make the band somewhat tight and then move the foot towards the ground, as seen below.

These exercises will strengthen the back of the leg, which contains the Achilles tendon and some of the other muscles that aid in moving the foot towards the ground. This movement is called plantar flexion.

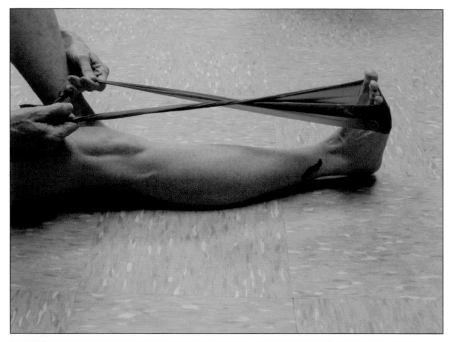

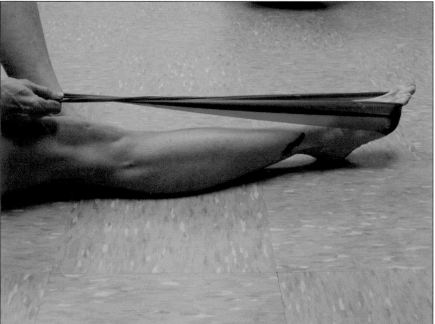

Push the foot down to strengthen the posterior muscles.

Strengthening the Intrinsic Muscles of the Foot

One aspect of strengthening that can be important to foot health is to improve the strength of the smallest muscle group in the feet (known as the intrinsic muscles because they start and end in the foot). These muscles are important to stability of the foot, and some experts think that weakness in the intrinsic muscles may be a contributing factor to plantar fasciitis and other foot ailments.

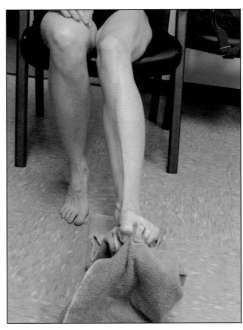

Use your toes to pick up a towel or t-shirt and hold it for a count of 5. Perform two sets of 15 repetitions.

Perform these exercises barefoot while sitting. They can be performed at various times throughout the day. Use a towel or shirt, and practice picking the item up with your toes and holding it for a count of five. Do 15 repetitions and complete two sets as part of your foot-strengthening circuit.

For the final exercise, place a book on the side of the towel farthest away from your foot. Use your toes to bunch up the towel or shirt and pull the book towards you. Perform 15 repetitions and complete two sets.

Arthur Lydiard, who is perhaps the greatest distance running coach ever, believed in the importance of strong feet. One of his quotes has always stuck with me: "You support an area [your foot], it gets weaker. Use it extensively, it gets stronger."

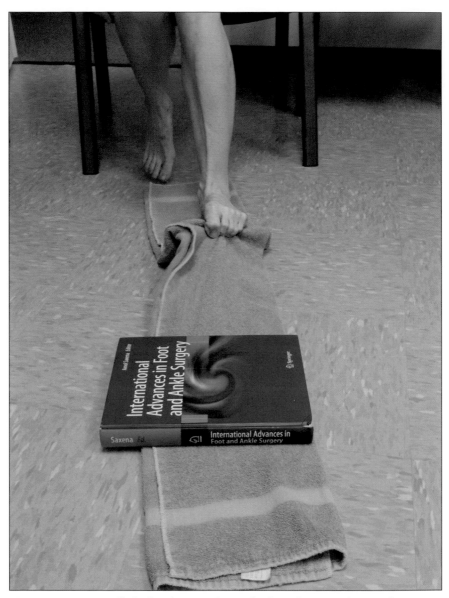

Use your toes to pull the book towards you by bunching up the towel. Perform two sets of 15 repetitions.

Chapter Seven

General Guidance on Injury Prevention

A major reason that preventing injury is so difficult is that we all respond differently to the stresses of training. While some runners can churn out 100 miles per week without ever sustaining a serious injury, others may get hurt running three miles a day.

That said, there are some general principles that runners should follow to lower their injury risk. Taking cautions such as gradually increasing training (some advocate not increasing your mileage by more than 10 percent per week), stretching on a routine basis, and incorporating planned easy days will almost certainly help you stay healthy and better able to meet your running goals. In this chapter, we'll look at preventative practices all runners can benefit from, as well as guidelines for finding a good sports medicine doctor if, unfortunately, you get injured.

Self-Monitoring and Self-Care

Keep a running log to help track how many miles you have on a pair of shoes. Most models will be past their peak efficiency after 300 to 500 miles. Some people will never see signs of wear on the outsole, but the midsole is the part of the shoe that breaks down and can lead to an injury if worn too long.

Respond to any swelling or pain by taking a rest day or two to see how the body responds. If pain persists past the first five minutes of a run, I advise not running, because if you're in pain you'll compensate for the injured body part, which can lead to injuries elsewhere. Use common sense and listen to your body—"rest" isn't always a bad, four-letter word.

Icing

The RICE method is commonly recommended for acute injuries such as an ankle sprain. The acronym stands for: R = rest, I = ice, C = compression, and E = elevation. Ice and compression have been found to help reduce pain and swelling. One high-level study found that 10 minutes was enough time to affect the temperature of the area being treated, and that pain and swelling were reduced better by alternating cooling and heating, repeated for three 10-minute icing sessions.

Ice can be used for chronic or acute injuries; tendons and joints will typically respond well to icing. If an area has swelling or is painful on a chronic basis, such as an arthritic knee or ankle, then ice can be a good choice. There's little downside from regular icing.

My recommendation is to use crushed ice or ice cubes with some water as opposed to reusable ice packs, which tend to be too cold initially but don't stay cold long enough. A thin towel can be placed between the skin and ice to help prevent a frostbite injury in certain areas that might be more sensitive to the cold, such as the top of the foot or outside of the knee.

Ice for 10 minutes at a time several times during the day. If you're treating an injury that's also swollen, add some compression with an ace bandage. If you are icing for iliotibial band syndrome on the side of the knee, it's very important to be mindful of not over-icing the common peroneal nerve in the area. A Major League Baseball player once iced his knee too long right over the nerve and ended up with a nerve injury that caused him to not be able to move his foot properly for a few days.

Active Warm-up

Medical studies have shown that static stretching of a muscle before an athletic activity can decrease the power and strength of that muscle. For this reason, an active warm-up is a much better choice before a run to improve your performance. There's also some evidence that a good warm-up might help to prevent injury.

Before a professional sporting event, you might see the athletes performing drills such as skipping or other exaggerated movements as part of an active warm-up. Gone are the days of the stretching circle before a practice, where you might have been told to

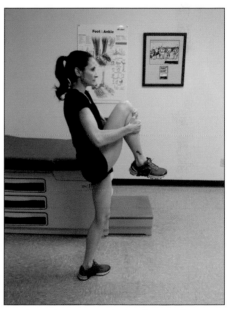

With each step, grab the front of your leg and pull up towards your body. Alternate each leg with each step and repeat 10 times for each leg.

"feel the burn" or "make it hurt" by trying to touch your toes to stretch your hamstrings.

There are several simple active warm-up exercises that can be performed in five minutes before your run. Active warm-up involves moving slowly through exaggerated movements. Perform 10 repetitions for each leg of each exercise right before you run.

Walk while doing all of these exercises. For the first, walk forward and, with each step, grab the front of your leg and pull it up to your body. This will help warm up the hip joints and hamstring muscles.

The next exercise integrates the upper body and targets the quadriceps muscles. With each step, grab your ankle and pull the foot to your butt while reaching to the sky with the opposite hand. Alternate legs, and do 10 times with each side.

The next exercise involves most of the lower leg in the form of walking lunges. Take as long of a step as possible and dip down into a lunge while keeping your back upright. Perform 10 repetitions on each leg.

Reach up to the sky with one hand, grab your foot with the opposite hand and pull it back. Try to pull your heel into your butt. Alternate feet for 10 repetitions.

The final exercise is straight leg kicks. Extend your leg in front of you, keeping your knee locked so that your leg is swinging from your hip. Raise the leg up as high as is comfortable. Do 10 with each leg. After completing this exercise you'll be better prepared to begin your run.

Stretching

Can stretching prevent injury? The short answer from the medical literature reveals minimal evidence that stretching can directly help to prevent an injury.

But there's difficulty in proving this hypothesis because other factors can contribute to an injury besides lack of flexibility. The best studies are prospective (which means the study begins before any results are known, whereas a retrospective study begins after the results of treatment are known) and double-blind (neither the researchers nor the subjects know who is getting which of the various experimental protocols). Known as level-1 studies, these investigations ideally provide an unbiased

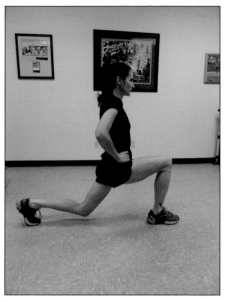

Walking lunges. Alternate each leg for 10 repetitions.

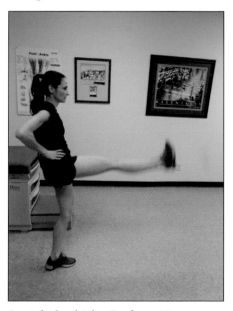

Straight leg kicks. Perform 10 steps with each leg.

viewpoint for what is being studied. Unfortunately, when doing a study on athletes to see if they get injured, it's difficult to control all the variables involved to prove that one aspect such as lack of stretching is to blame.

There are definitely benefits to stretching—it's been shown to improve joint mobility and range of motion. Stretching should never be painful. Stretching should be performed after you run, as it's much easier to safely stretch a muscle that's warm.

There are many methods of stretching, including active isolated (popularized in running by Jim and Phil Wharton), ballistic and, the simplest, static. All are proven to improve flexibility. While you'll find passionate adherents for each type, I think the most important thing is to use whichever method you'll do regularly.

Below are three simple stretches that will help maintain your flexibility and range of motion. I recommend doing them regularly after your runs.

Calf Stretching

Every runner can benefit from stretching the calf muscles. In addition to helping with calf flexibility, this stretch will increase ankle joint mobility, which has been proven to be important to proper form and function of the rest of the body.

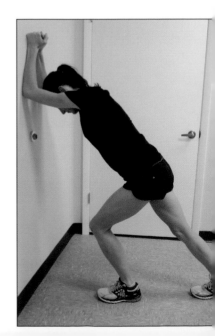

Proper form for the wall stretch. Hold for 30 seconds and repeat three times (five if you're injured), alternating legs.

Static stretching is the safest to perform. Static means that you stretch the muscle until a good tension is felt and then you hold it without any bouncing or other movements.

Keep your back foot flat on the ground and lean in until you feel a good pull in your calf muscles. You shouldn't feel pain or discomfort. Hold the stretch for 30 seconds per leg, and repeat three times for each leg. Do the stretch five times if you have a lower-leg injury such as plantar fasciitis or medial tibial stress syndrome (shin splints).

Hamstring Stretching

The hamstring muscles in the back of the thigh are often tight and/or sore from running. Maintaining flexibility in this group can help improve your performance. If the hamstring muscles tighten, you'll have a shorter stride.

It's important to note that you never want a muscle to be active while you're stretching it. So for a stretch of the hamstring, it's best if the leg is supported (avoid putting your foot up on a bench or railing as the nerve can be stretched and damaged). Keep your back straight as well. There's no need to try to touch your toes. Just lean forward until you feel the tension of a good pull in your hamstring. This stretch

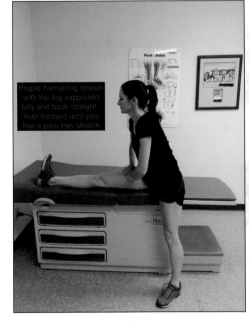

This stretch can also be performed on the ground. Keep your back straight and lean forward with your entire torso. Hold the stretch for 30 seconds, switch legs, and repeat three times.

can also be performed on the ground. Keep your back straight and lean forward with your entire torso until you feel a good stretch in your hamstrings.

Gluteal and Piriformis Stretching

The piriformis is a muscle below the all-important gluteal muscles. A tight piriformis can irritate the sciatic nerve and cause pain down the leg, including when sitting. The gluteal muscles will also benefit from this stretch.

Lie on your back and cross one leg over the other above the knee as seen below. Grab the leg that's not crossed over and pull it towards your chest. You'll feel the stretch in the buttocks area. Hold for 30 seconds and alternate legs for three stretches on each side.

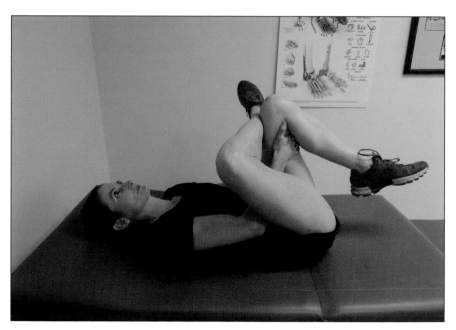

Cross one leg over the other, grab the opposite leg and pull it towards your chest. Hold the stretch for 30 seconds and alternate legs three times.

Yoga

Yoga can be a great way for runners to improve their flexibility and balance. Some people benefit from taking a class while others can do it at home. Yoga enthusiasts tout the benefits of improved balance, lengthened muscles (which will, in turn, improve range of motion), and increased strength.

Pilates

Joseph Pilates was a physical trainer from Germany who developed the basic principles of the exercises that bear his name. Pilates shares some similarities with yoga but is more focused on strengthening the core muscles, which are so important to the runner. There are Pilates studios with the special equipment that can be used for this exercise, but the movements can be done at home without any special equipment.

Two Dietary Matters

A good diet is an important part of overall health. For our purposes here, we'll focus on two nutrients, vitamin D and calcium, that both have a strong bearing on common running injuries.

Vitamin D is critical to bone health and has also been found to help with muscle function, recovery from workouts and injuries, and the body's immunity to fight off infections and sickness. It's more than a vitamin; the body metabolizes it to become similar to a steroid.

Normal blood values for vitamin D are above 30 nmol/L, but for athletes the optimal number may actually be over 75. When you have routine blood work done, ask to have your vitamin D levels checked; you might be deficient but unaware of it. For example, I found out that my level was 9 in a recent blood test. That probably happened because, as a resident of Florida, I always wear sunscreen, and an SPF of 15 will block 95 percent of the body's ability to produce vitamin D from sun exposure. Some experts suggest 15 minutes a day of sun exposure without sun block, preferably midday to achieve suitable levels of vitamin D.

Two recent studies highlight the importance of vitamin D to bone health. The first showed that, in Finnish military recruits, stress fracture risk was 3.6 times higher in those with relatively low vitamin D status (< 75 nmol/L) compared to those with higher status. Another high-level study of vitamin D3 supplementation (daily 800 IU with 2 g calcium) found a 20 percent reduction in stress fracture incidence in female U.S. Navy recruits compared to those taking a placebo.

The sun is the best source of Vitamin D production; aim for 15 minutes a day with arms, face, and legs exposed. If you live in area where consistent sun exposure isn't possible, supplementation is a good idea; 1,000 IUs a day is usually a safe dosage.

Dietary sources of vitamin D include salmon, sardines, tuna, shiitake mushrooms, egg yolks, cheese, and milk. Many foods are fortified with vitamin D, which is better than taking a supplement.

Calcium is very important to bone health. Dietary intake should be 1,000 to 1,200 mg per day. Our bodies absorb it best from food. Dairy products along with green leafy vegetables have the highest amount of calcium. Well-absorbable plant-based calcium can be found in lettuce, celery or spinach, fortified juices, soy milk or meat, rice milk, and certain legumes (e.g., soybeans and peanuts). Sardines are also an excellent nondairy source of absorbable calcium.

For those who are unable to meet their calcium requirements from food sources, calcium supplementation of 1,000 mg/day is recommended, particularly in women with menstrual irregularities. It's best to take the pills in two doses of 500 mg, one in the morning and one at night. Calcium carbonate and calcium citrate are the most well absorbed sources used in supplements.

How to Choose the Right Doctor

Unfortunately, even if you do everything the right way, you might be injured. (Some studies report that half of all runners will experience an injury at some point.)

Choosing the right doctor to see can prove to be a challenge. It can seem like almost every podiatrist, chiropractor, physical therapist, and orthopedist lists sports medicine as one of their specialties, but not all are truly practicing with athletes' best interests in mind.

My simple definition of "sports medicine" mirrors my idea of the best way to treat every patient: sports medicine professionals have a duty to the patient to make a proper diagnosis and treat the cause of the injury, not just the symptoms.

A sports medicine specialist should have the mindset of trying every treatment possible that's medically proven in order to return athletes to their desired sport and activity level as quickly and safely as possible. The physician should almost never tell their athletic patients not to work out or to give up their sport of choice without a valid reason or a timetable for future treatments and testing. There should always be several plans laid out, as many times there are multiple potential differential diagnoses at work.

Athletes are typically well-informed patients. Ideally, they're given credit for this knowledge by their physician and are allowed to properly collaborate in their treatment. Use PubMed.org when researching your condition. It's an excellent resource for reading abstracts and articles about almost any topic that's published in a peer-reviewed medical journal. It's important to look critically at every study—consider the level of evidence-based medicine and see who supported the funding of the study. Be wary of press releases touting an article in the lay press.

How do physicians arrive at a good diagnosis? The best start is a thorough history. Patients should leave no stone unturned in relating the course of their injury, because there are always clues that might be a key to putting the puzzle together. It's so important for the physician to listen to the patient and try not to interrupt. In a study from the University of South Carolina, on average doctors interrupted patients within eleven seconds, and often didn't allow patients to finish their sentences. The average encounter was eleven minutes, with patients speaking for only four minutes of that time.

The patient should expect the doctor to place their hands on the patient to palpate the injured area, check ranges of motion, and watch the patient walk and/or run, if possible. There's certainly a place for tests such as an X-ray, MRI, CT Scan, bone scan, and diagnostic ultrasound. But patient and doctor alike should be asking themselves this question: Will the new test help make a diagnosis and will it change my treatment plan? For example, for diagnosing a Morton's neuroma, research shows that clinical diagnosis is equal to diagnostic ultrasound and superior to an MRI. A recent paper found a squeeze test between forefinger and thumb to be the best test. Tests aren't always necessary, and for many patients can be a significant financial burden.

A negative test doesn't always mean there's nothing wrong. In the past two years I've treated two runners with leg pain who had negative MRIs and radiographs from other doctors. Both exhibited stress fracture-like symptoms, and both tested positive for that injury when I had them undergo a triphasic bone scan, a sometimes forgotten-about diagnostic test.

As a patient, don't be satisfied with a negative X-ray or MRI in the presence of symptoms; very seldom does a problem or injury exist only in your mind. I can't recall a single athletic patient who did not want to get better. If your doctor has failed to arrive at a diagnosis after several office visits and tests, change your view of the injury, think of what other possible causes exist, and never be afraid to ask for another opinion from a different physician.

If you have an important competition in the near future, you should expect your doctor to offer a more aggressive treatment program, if the injury lends itself to this possibility. The sports medicine professional must understand that a college athlete has only four years of eligibility, a high school athlete may be trying to win a college scholarship, or an adult runner might be preparing for a once-in-a-lifetime run at an event like the Boston Marathon.

Of course, you and your doctor must temper that aggressiveness if there's a possibility of long-term harm. It can be a difficult dilemma. Recently I treated a runner with pain in a muscle one month before a championship race. The athlete wanted me to inject cortisone. I advised the patient that a complete rupture was possible, and I asked if she planned to continue racing professionally after the championship. Her affirmative response led me to deny the injection. An MRI revealed a muscle tear, at which point no running was an important part of recovery.

How Do You Know if You're in the Wrong Doctor's Office?

There are several red flags for the athlete/patient that they might be in the wrong office. The biggest one for a runner is if the physician makes a comment such as "running is bad for you."

Another is being put in a boot for an extended period of time and/or being told not to run without a diagnosis. For the athlete, every day in that boot adds another day you have to strengthen the area that's immobilized after the boot is removed. I once treated the captain of a Division I college cross country team who had been given a diagnosis of metatarsalgia, which is a general term for pain in the front of the foot. The school's sports medicine staff had the athlete in a short leg walking cast boot for the six weeks before his visit to my office. It turned out the runner was suffering from a neuroma, and after a single corticosteroid injection and a pad in the shoe he was back to running. But he had missed his last season of collegiate eligibility because of a misdiagnosis and the consequent time in the boot.

Also be suspicious when you're asked to return multiple times to the office for treatments and tests that can and should be performed in one visit. If an X-ray is taken, it should be reviewed during that visit, not dangled as a carrot to try to capture another co-pay and office visit from the patient. Some doctors see dollar signs when an athlete such as a runner or triathlete walks in the door. Custom orthotic devices are not a cure-all for every ailment, and some patients are wrongly placed in devices that aren't necessary. Patients shouldn't be afraid to question a treatment plan, which should be a collaborative effort.

Chapter Eight
When to Seek Surgery

This chapter will highlight some of the more common foot surgeries that a runner might be forced to consider and help guide the choice of the proper procedure.

When deciding whether surgery makes sense, here's an important question to answer: Have you exhausted more conservative treatments that will cure your problem instead of just treating its symptoms? The best person to answer these questions with you is your local sports podiatrist. Ideally, you want your podiatrist to be both a fellow of the American Academy of Podiatric Sports Medicine (aapsm.org) and board-certified in foot surgery by The American Board of Podiatric Surgery (abps.org). As we'll see, there are times when surgery should be considered as something other than your last resort.

Choosing an experienced surgeon who is board-certified in foot surgery is extremely important. You can search abfas.org/findadoctor for a qualified surgeon. The ABPS certifies qualified podiatrists in foot surgery and also ankle surgery. The process involves taking written and oral examinations to attain board-certified status, which must be renewed every ten years with new tests to ensure surgeons are up-to-date on best practices. Once you've found a surgeon, keep in mind that sometimes it's worth the effort to obtain a second opinion from another qualified surgeon. If a doctor is unable to answer questions about return to activity or doesn't consider your running and activity level when choosing a surgical procedure, then seek another opinion from a podiatrist who is more sports-oriented.

Other factors for runners to consider: some surgeries are easier to recover from than others, and the best surgery for most patients may not be the best for an athlete. A good example is the choice of surgery to correct a bunion deformity. One of the more effective and popular surgeries performed now is called a Lapidus, which involves fusing the joint at the apex of the deformity known as the first metatarsal-cuneiform joint. In my opinion, fusions of joints should be avoided in athletes if at all possible. Once a joint is fused, the adjacent joints will start to break down sooner and the foot doesn't function the same once motion is removed from any joint.

Paula Radcliffe, the women's world record holder in the marathon, first noticed pain from a bunion after she won the 2005 world championships marathon. Over the next four years, she suffered a series of injuries, and despite occasional bright spots, such as winning the 2007 and 2008 runnings of the New York City Marathon, she was in rehab more often than not. Finally, in May 2009, Radcliffe underwent bunion surgery by a podiatrist. A surgeon who was not as experienced in working with athletes may have viewed the X-rays and extent of the deformity and performed a more aggressive correction, possibly a Lapidus.

"When we sat down and looked at my injury history prior to the surgery in 2009, we realized that every injury, bar one,

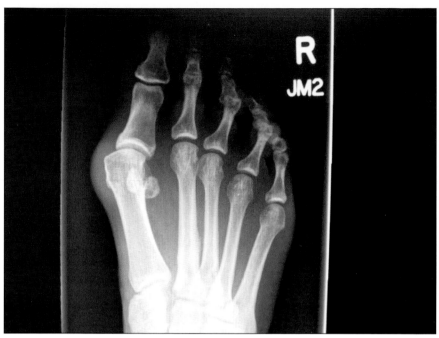

Paula Radcliffe's pre-op X-rays. Note the protrusion of the first metatarsal away from the second metatarsal.

Image courtesy of Dr. Amol Saxena

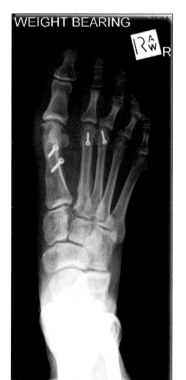

Dr. Amol Saxena performed a surgery on Radcliffe without fusing any joints to correct the deformity.

Image courtesy of Dr. Amol Saxena

since 2004 had been caused directly or indirectly by the bunion," Radcliffe said. "Even the femoral stress fracture was related to my bunion pain, as it came from imbalances caused by modifying my orthotics to enable me to run on the right foot without significant pain."

Could Radcliffe have returned to normal running sooner by taking the counterintuitive step of opting for surgery earlier? While foot surgery should usually be considered a last resort after conservative treatment has failed, there are times when surgery may allow a runner to return to training faster. As in Radcliffe's case, surgery can often provide a cure, while conservative treatment may only be treating the symptoms. Surgical techniques have improved considerably in the last decade; advances that allow for faster recovery and more predictable results can mean that the runner's traditional avoidance of surgery is based on outdated thinking.

Let's look at some of the common foot injuries and deformities that are operated on—bunions, hammer toes, neuromas, Achilles tendon problems, and plantar fasciitis—in terms of when to consider surgery over more conservative treatment. First, though, these caveats: You should always understand that there aren't any guarantees with any surgical procedure. Even the best surgeon in the world has poor outcomes. It's also important to note that some people take longer than average to heal, while some can return to activity faster.

Bunions

The medical term for a bunion is hallux abducto valgus (HAV), which indicates that the hallux (big toe) deviates towards the second toe, and the first metatarsal head protrudes in the opposite direction. The most common complaint associated with this deformity is pain at the medial (inner) aspect of the joint.

The deformity is commonly considered an inherited trait. There's no scientific evidence that a bunion can be prevented with any treatments, but the pain and symptoms can be managed.

Conservative treatment starts with making sure your shoes are wide enough. A good brand to try before considering surgery is Altra, which features a foot-shaped toe box that allows plenty of the room for the forefoot. Occasionally treatments such as cortisone injections, custom orthotic devices, and various paddings and splints can help to treat the symptoms, but surgery is the only option to correct this problem.

I don't recommend surgical correction unless you have pain that severely limits your running and/or daily activities. But bear in mind that, as in Radcliffe's case, some injuries elsewhere may be indirectly related to the lack of proper function of the big toe joint due to HAV.

Surgical correction typically involves cutting and repositioning the first metatarsal with the use of screws, plates, or pins to hold the bone in the proper position while it heals. Depending on the severity of the deformity, the bone may need to be cut at different spots. The severity of the bunion determines what procedure is required; larger deformities require more extensive correction, leading to a longer recovery time. Expect to miss a minimum of six to eight weeks; for some procedures, up to sixteen weeks of time off from running will be required.

The use of newer and better screws has shortened the recovery time considerably. Some screws have a lower profile, which often eliminates any discomfort associated with the head of the screw and allows the screw to remain in place permanently. For some procedures, removal of screws or other hardware after bone healing is complete is considered on a routine basis.

Bunion deformities are divided into mild, moderate and severe, and are based on physical appearance as well as what's seen in X-rays. Angles can be drawn over X-ray images to help the doctor determine which procedure is appropriate.

One of the more important angles is called the Inter-metatarsal Angle, or IM angle, between the first and second metatarsals. It measures the amount of distance that the first metatatarsal is moving away from the second. The greater the IM angle, the farther away from the big toe joint the first metatarsal needs to be cut and shifted. In many cases, if the IM angle is below 15 degrees, then a simpler procedure can be performed, making recovery and return to running easier.

If the first metatarsal is cut closer to the base, then non-weight bearing in a short leg cast will be required for up to four to six weeks. The Lapidus procedure further adds to the difficulty in healing by using a fusion of two bones at the first metatarsal, the cuneiform joint. The medical literature points out that up to 10 percent of Lapidus procedures will have a non-union of the fusion. This means up to an added two to six months of either casting to allow the union to take place, sometimes with the addition of a bone stimulator, or the need for a second surgery involving bone grafting and further alteration of the mechanics of the foot. Placing the Lapidus in the proper position while fusing is another complication—the first metatarsal can

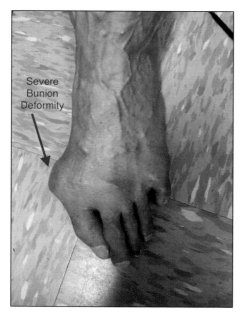

Severe
Bunion
Deformity

A severe bunion.

end up too elevated or too plantarflexed (in a position lower than the other bones). If the first metatarsal is too elevated that places the patient at risk for a stress fracture in the lesser metatarsals. If the bone is too plantarflexed then the sesamoids or other structures around the big toe joint may be put under too much stress.

An Austin bunionectomy is one of the more common procedures performed. It involves a V-shaped osteotomy (cutting and shifting of the bone) that allows the first metatarsal head to be shifted back towards the second metatarsal. The hallux will then move away from the second toe into a more normal position in which the first metatarsal joint (MPJ) will then be more congruent (lined up properly). When the joint is out of place, it can lead to degenerative changes in the cartilage of the first MPJ, making motion painful with every step in severe cases.

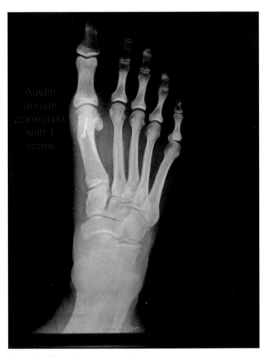

Austin bunion correction.

There are dozens of different surgical procedures to correct a bunion deformity. Discuss with your surgeon the different options including the recovery time and possible side effects that will impact your future running.

Tailor's Bunion

The fifth metatarsal can deviate laterally, on the opposite side of an HAV deformity, causing pain and difficulty in finding shoes that fit. In this condition, there appears to be bowing out

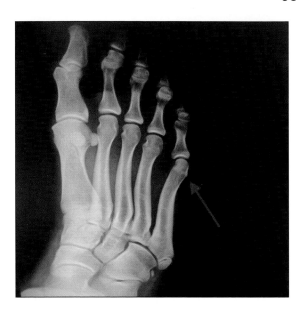

Tailor's bunion X-ray.

of the bone. Other than choosing wider shoes, there's not a lot of conservative treatment to help alleviate the symptoms of this deformity if it has progressed to a painful condition.

If the pain is significant enough to cause you to limit your activity, then surgery can help eliminate the pain. Surgery entails cutting the bone and shifting it towards the inside of the foot, and placing a screw through the bone cut. Expect returning to running to take at least six to eight weeks with a normal course of healing.

Hallux Limitus

In the late 1980s and early 1990s, John Trautmann was one of the brightest stars in American distance running. In 1986, he broke the legendary Steve Prefontaine's high school 3,000-meter record, and followed that with an accomplished collegiate career at Georgetown University. As a professional, John won the 1992 U.S. Olympic Trials in the 5,000 meters.

But John had trouble competing in Barcelona in the 1992 Olympics because of plantar fasciitis and Achilles tendinosis. His troubles were eventually found to stem from a lack of motion in the big toe joint, a condition known as hallux limitus.

To combat this, John underwent two less-than-successful surgeries to try to alleviate his pain and improve the function

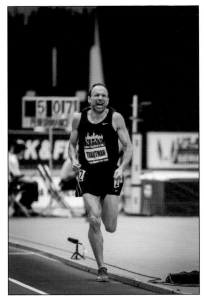

John Trautmann as a masters runner.

Photo by Joe Navas

of his first metatarsal phalangeal joint (MPJ). He eventually had the big toe joint fused and quit running. At age forty, John began running again to lose weight, and at the age of forty-six ran a 4:12 mile, a world record for his age group.

The fusion isn't the ideal procedure for a runner, but in John's case it was performed because he had pain during his activities of daily living and at the time he was not planning on competing at a high level anymore. The surgery allows him to run pain-free, but John knows that he's compensating for the fused joint.

The big toe is known as the hallux. It must form an angle with the first metatarsal head of at least 45 degrees for proper toe-off. If that motion is limited, compensation will occur that can affect everything up to the back.

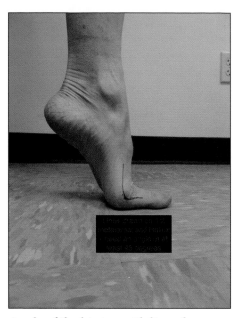

Angle of the big toe with lines drawn.

Motion can be limited in a functional or structural manner; the type of limitation is important in determining the best treatment. In a functional hallux limitus, there's enough range of motion when the foot isn't in contact with the ground, but when the foot is in what's known as a loaded position at toe-off, the first metatarsal head will elevate enough to cause a jamming effect of the first metatarsal phalangeal joint. The result is less-than-desirable motion. Over time, if there's repetitive jamming in the joint a bone spur may develop on the top of the first metatarsal head and lead to a more structural problem. The jamming at the end range of motion also causes a compressive force on the first metatarsal head and leads to destruction of the cartilage.

Hallux limitus has a commonly accepted grading schedule, with Grade 1 being more of a functional limitation of motion, Grades 2 and 3 involve more and more damage to the joint cartilage, with less motion as the deformity progresses. If untreated, the final stage is Grade 4, hallux rigidus, at which point there's no motion occurring in the big toe joint due to severe arthritis and loss of cartilage.

Conservative treatment revolves around inserts for shoes and different shoes being used. A simple solution is to add extra padding under the big toe joint. This is called a Morton's

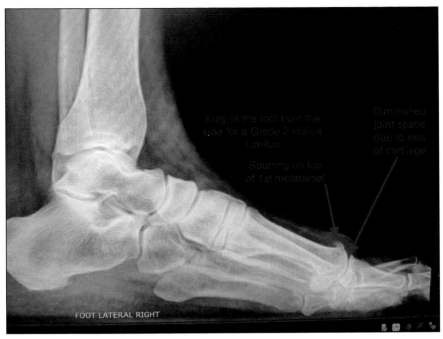

X-ray of hallux limitus, Stage 1 or 2.

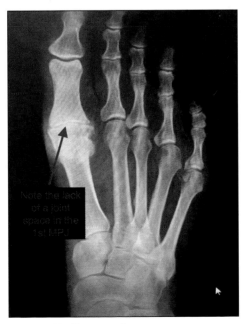

X-ray of hallux rigidus.

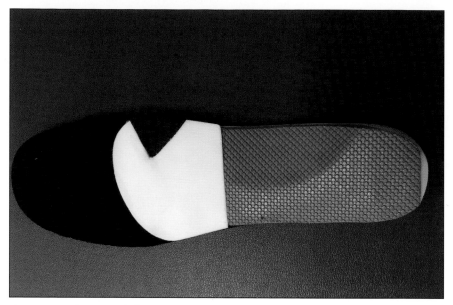

Custom orthotic with kinetic wedge.

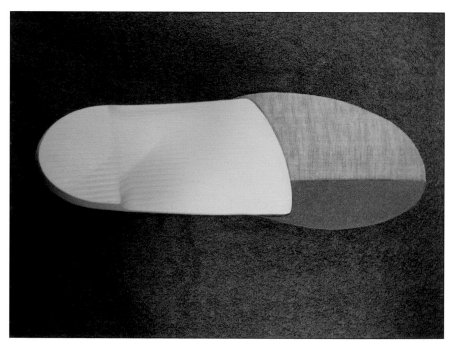

Orthotic with Morton's extension.

extension, and splints the first MPJ to take some of the pressure off the area. I sometimes add 1/8" of cork to the bottom of the sockliner of a running shoe or to an over-the-counter arch support. If the Morton's extension doesn't work, then I switch to a reverse Morton's or Kinetic Wedge-type device, which features a cutout under the first metatarsal to allow it to drop lower and give the first MPJ to more relative dorsiflexion.

There are four basic types of surgeries that are performed on the first MPJ for hallux limitus and rigidus. One study found similar satisfaction rates across all four types of procedures, but the patient population was not athletic.

The simplest procedure removes a portion of the top of the first metatarsal head. The least aggressive of these types of procedures is called a cheilectomy, which involves removing the spurring at the top of the joint. If there are defects in the cartilage of the first metatarsal head, then holes can be drilled in the metatarsal head during the surgery to promote the growth of new cartilage. The new cartilage is known as fibrocartilage, which isn't as good as the normal cartilage, but it's better than not having any cartilage at all in the area.

A more aggressive type of procedure similar to the cheilectomy is called a Valenti procedure. More of the bone is removed from the top of the first metatarsal head and some of the bone is removed from the base of the proximal phalanx, the toe bone that makes up part of the joint along with the metatarsal heal. Several prominent surgeons now use this procedure extensively in even the most severe deformities with great success in athletes.

The next type of procedure involves cutting and shifting the bone. The goal is to shorten and lower the first metatarsal head to attempt to create more space in the big toe joint and reposition the joint to take advantage of better cartilage. One type of this procedure is a modified Austin-type bone cut that places a single screw at the osteotomy site. I have performed this successfully on many runners and continue to use this and the modified Valenti as my procedures of choice.

The next two surgical procedures for hallux limitus are called joint destructive procedures. One uses a joint replacement implant and the other fuses the joint. There are different types of implants, but that surgery isn't one that I would ever recommend for a runner, because running will lead to the implant breaking down sooner. Fusions should only be considered as a last resort or a salvage procedure, as in John Trautmann's case, where he already had two prior surgeries performed on the joint. If, for whatever reason, a fusion doesn't allow normal activity, then there's very little that can be done to rectify the problem. So don't enter into that choice of procedure lightly.

Neuromas

A neuroma is inflammation of the nerve in the ball of the foot, most commonly involving the area between the second and third metatarsal heads or the third and fourth metatarsal heads. Symptoms include pain in the area directly before the toes, shooting pain into the toes, numbness in the area, and sometimes a feeling of walking on a marble.

The majority of the time, conservative treatment, consisting of wider or more cushioned shoes, custom orthotic devices, cortisone injections, and padding around the area, can alleviate the pain. One last resort before considering surgical intervention is a series of injections using a 4 percent solution of alcohol mixed with local anesthetic, a procedure known as sclerotherapy. The alcohol causes degeneration of the nerve fibers. The protocol involves a series of three to seven injections performed weekly. One study reported an 89 percent success rate with the procedure. I've not found anywhere close to that level of success, but there are no apparent negative side effects to sclerotherapy.

One runner I treated tried all of the above, including sclerotherapy, to deal with pain in her foot that was bad enough to interfere with her training. When none of the conservative treatments brought relief, she elected to undergo surgical excision of the nerve. Like most foot surgery, hers was performed on an outpatient basis. She was running within four weeks of her surgery. Several years later, she's still pain-free at her former neuroma location.

A simpler technique involves cutting the ligament that runs over the top of the nerve. Neuromas are close to the base of the toes, which have a ligament on the top and bottom. The theory is that this "decompresses" the nerve, thereby relieving the pain.

Dr. Michael Chin, one of the medical directors of the Chicago Marathon, inspects the nerve for damage during surgery. After cutting the ligament on the top of the nerve, he makes the decision whether to remove the diseased portion of the nerve or to just reposition it. If the nerve appears normal (scar tissue around the nerve turns the nerve tissue yellow, while a healthy nerve is white and glistening), then Dr. Chin will use a hammock technique with suture material to raise the nerve slightly above the level of the metatarsals to relieve the pain. There's little downside to this procedure. If pain persists after this surgery, then the nerve can be excised in the traditional manner.

Achilles Tendon Surgery

Achilles tendinitis is one of the more difficult injuries any athlete can encounter. Within two weeks of Achilles inflammation, the tendon fibers begin to degenerate. After exhausting all conservative treatments, then surgery can be considered in some cases. (See Chapter 4 for much more on Achilles injuries.)

If the problem is due to the paratenon (the sheath that covers the tendon), then the surgery simply involves making an incision in this sheath and cutting the scarred portion of the paratenon away from the Achilles. An athlete may be able to return to training within a month after this surgery. Surgery for Achilles pain on the tendon in the mid substance involves cutting out the degenerated portion of the tendon and repairing the remaining tendon on either side of the defect with suture material.

Pain that's closer to the attachment of the Achilles in the back of the calcaneus (heel bone), where patients may commonly have a bone spur, is known as a Haglund's deformity. The use of anchors has further enhanced surgery involving the back of the heel, allowing the tendon to be detached to remove any bone spurring, and then reattached with the use of an anchor. Recovery involves being in a short leg cast initially, then a removable cast followed by physical therapy, with a return to running in roughly three months. World championships marathoner Keith Dowling had pain for the last two years of his competitive career from a Haglund's deformity. After failed conservative treatment I operated on Keith using anchors. He doesn't compete anymore but is able to run with no pain in the back of his heel.

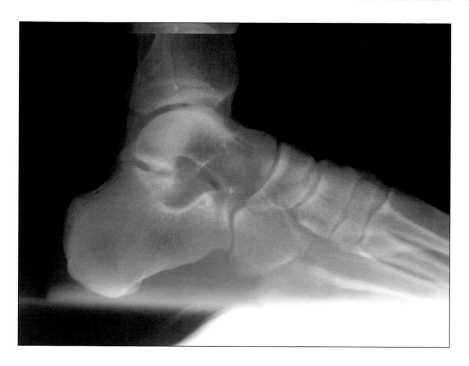

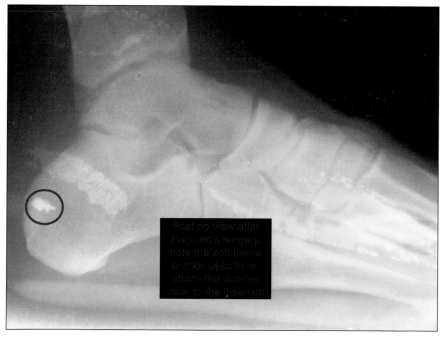

Post op view after
Haglund's surgery,
note the soft tissue
anchor used to re-
attach the achilles
back to the insertion

Keith Dowling's heel before and after.

Plantar Fascial Surgery

This injury typically resolves more than 90 percent of the time with conservative treatment. The most important factor in treating this very common injury is early intervention. Calf stretching, icing with a frozen water bottle 20 to 30 minutes two or three times per day, taping and massage are the initial treatments, and work well for up to half of patients with this injury. When those treatments don't help, then cortisone injections, over-the-counter and custom orthotic devices are the next level of conservative management.

Shock wave therapy has been found to resolve plantar fasciitis in up 70 percent of cases that didn't improve with more conventional treatments. It's crucial that your physician rule out other causes of heel pain, such as nerve entrapment, before considering surgery; often an MRI should be ordered to confirm the proper diagnosis.

There are several surgical approaches, including endoscopic plantar fasciotomy, in which the fascia is cut at the insertion point; ideally there's minimal trauma to the tissue due to the use of arthroscopy. A traditional open approach allows the surgeon to examine for nerve entrapment, but it involves a larger incision, creating the possibility of more scar tissue, which can, ironically, cause nerve entrapment.

Another approach, known as an instep fasciotomy, involves making the incision right in the arch on the bottom of the foot over the area where the fascia will be cut. This procedure has the advantage of causing less scar tissue. The post-op course should involve at least a three-week period of no weight bearing to allow the cut portion of the plantar fascia to fill in with scar tissue, which essentially leads to an elongated ligament and less tension on the fascia, and should alleviate the pain of this injury.

The most worrisome complication involves creating instability of the foot by severing the entire plantar fascia across the bottom of the foot. Most surgeons won't cut the fascia completely; they often leave the outside portion of the fascia intact, cutting only about 75 percent of the way across the fascia. Calcaneal cuboid syndrome, which leads to severe pain on the outside of the foot, is one possible complication that can be extremely difficult to resolve. Of all the surgeries in the foot, this is the one that should absolutely be considered as the last resort.

Hammer Toes

Hammer toe is a deformity that leads to a portion of the toe sticking up and rubbing on the shoe. Sometimes a callus will form and become painful with any pressure on the area; this is commonly called a corn.

Conservative treatment starts with the simplest change of a deeper toe box. Padding can be applied to the toe, and shaving of the corn can sometimes relieve a lot of the symptoms.

In severe cases, surgery can be performed. The simplest procedure involves removing a small piece of bone from one of the three bones in the digit, the proximal phalanx. This is called an arthroplasty. There are a variety of other techniques done to help correct a hammer toe, including fusing the joint where the arthroplasty is performed or stabilizing the area with a removable pin or absorbable pin. A minimum of four weeks will be required before returning to running (longer if a fusion is attempted).

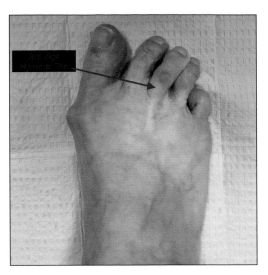

A hammer toe.

In an advanced stage, you might have pain under the metatarsal head, because as the hammer toe gets worse the proximal phalanx will displace to a position more on top of the metatarsal, forcing the metatarsal down and creating more pressure and pain in the ball of the foot.

The plantar plate, a structure that aids in maintaining the normal alignment of all our toes, is at the bottom of the joint. The plantar plate is a thin piece of cartilage-like material that attaches to the underside of the proximal phalanx. When placed under repetitive stress the plantar plate can tear, and if the damage progresses to a complete tear then the toe will dislocate.

Surgery to repair a plantar plate tear involves repairing the hammer toe and then cutting the metatarsal to shorten the bone to reduce the pressure on the area, followed by repairing the plantar plate to stabilize the toe. If the metatarsal bone is cut and repositioned, then expect a minimum of eight weeks before returning to activity.

Surgery on any part of the foot or ankle is a serious undertaking. I highly recommend that all conservative treatment be exhausted before considering surgery. Even if the surgery looks perfect afterwards there may still be pain, which can impact any activity. Weigh the risks versus the benefits and make an educated decision based on discussion with your podiatrist.

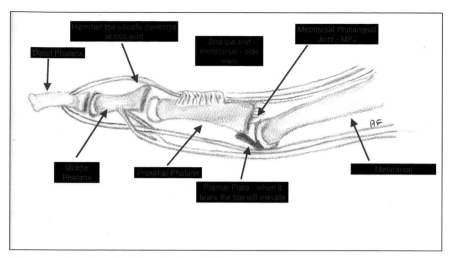

Hammer toe showing the plantar plate.

Drawing by Annemarie Fullem, PT.

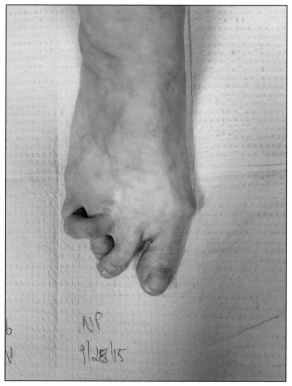

A dislocated toe.

Chapter Nine

New Treatments and Technologies

Technology has produced some great advances in equipment for runners to use for running and cross training as well as in the medical treatment of injured athletes. In this chapter we'll review some of the best new tools that can help a runner stay healthy or, if injured, allow a faster return to activity.

Extracorporeal Shockwave Therapy (ESWT)

Throughout this book I've highlighted this therapy as a good way to treat many running injuries. The technology was first applied to break up kidney stones in 1980 and was called lithotripsy. In the years since it's found a great number of applications for many different types of injuries. The units have become smaller and are now able to be offered in doctors' offices.

The devices use a hand-held piece that delivers strong sound waves deep into the tissue. The initial devices were very painful and required a nerve block around the ankle to numb the entire foot before treatment. Modern devices are able to deliver the sound waves with a tolerable amount of discomfort. Studies have shown that using a local anesthetic to numb the area prior to treatment leads to worse outcomes.

A series of three to five treatments spaced one to two weeks apart has become a normal protocol. Some of the newer devices are known as radial shockwave (r-EWST), the difference being that these units don't penetrate as deeply as ESWT, but in the foot and leg there's no need to penetrate any deeper. The medical literature doesn't reveal much of a difference in the efficacy of the two types of ESWT.

The technology helps to produce new blood supply to the area, leading to enhanced healing of soft-tissue injuries such as plantar fasciitis, Achilles tendonitis, and most other tendon pathologies. It's currently being studied for nerve pain. There's substantial evidence that ESWT can also help fractures heal better. The possibilities are endless because the technology is completely safe without any significant side effects. A recent medical report identified ESWT as the platinum standard for heel pain. Some studies report up to an 80 percent success rate for eliminating pain in the heel and Achilles.

The Verdict: The best treatment currently available for heel pain, plantar fasciitis, and most tendinopathies in the feet and ankles, including the Achilles, peroneal tendons, and posterior tibial tendons. It's worth using to help fractures heal quicker and for other injuries such sesamoid injuries and neuromas. The best feature is that there's no damage to the area treated. The worst result is that it may not help.

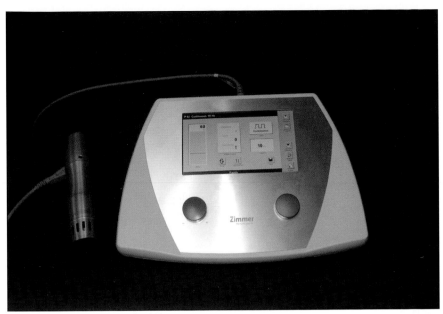

Radial Extracorporeal Shockwave unit made by Zimmer Medizin Systems. The treatment area is covered in mineral oil and the hand piece delivers the sound waves into the area.

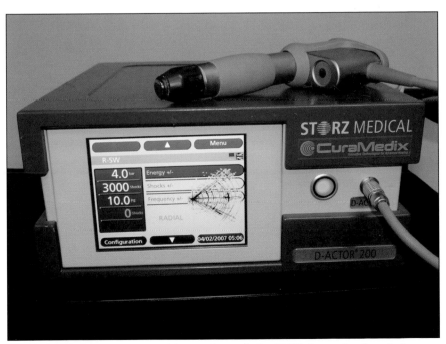

Storz Medical D-Actor 200 delivers the radial ESWT through a hand piece to the injured tissue.

Platelet Rich Plasma (PRP)

PRP is a treatment involving giving a sample of your own blood, which is then processed in a centrifuge to extract the plasma that's injected into the injured tendon or muscle. The treatment is often used on high-level athletes and is often touted in the media for its great healing powers.

The treatment is costly and not covered by insurance, and scientific studies haven't shown it to be any more effective than a placebo. In a review of all the medical studies on the use of PRP, the authors found just three high-quality studies among all the literature published, and none of these studies showed any statistically significant improvement compared to a placebo.

The Verdict: There's no harm from this treatment, and the potential as a viable treatment makes sense given the potential healing properties of the platelets. But I wouldn't spend a significant amount of money on this unproven treatment until better evidence is shown in the medical literature.

Dry Needling

Dry needling is used for soft-tissue pain associated with trigger points, those knots you might sometimes feel in your muscles. Massage therapy and active release technique are two traditional ways to break up trigger points; doing so is thought to reduce pain and allow the associated muscle and tendon to function better.

Dry needling uses monofilament needles similar to acupuncture needles, which are inserted into the trigger point areas. The medical literature reveals good short-term outcomes at reducing pain without any long-term benefits.

The Verdict: Not a first-line or stand-alone treatment, but if offered by an experienced practitioner it could help to reduce your pain in the short term.

Prolotherapy

Prolotherapy is a treatment offered for tendon, ligament, and joint injuries in which dextrose (a sugar solution) is injected into the area. The thought is that the dextrose leads the body to have an inflammatory reaction, the response to which helps the damaged tissue be repaired.

The introduction of a needle (which is much thicker than those used in acupuncture or dry needling) may be the reason for the traumatic reaction. The medical literature shows no difference in most studies between this treatment and a placebo.

The Verdict: Avoid this treatment.

Radiofrequency Nerve Ablation

Nerve ablation is a minimally invasive surgical procedure. The technique involves inserting a needle-like probe into the area of a nerve thought to be causing pain such as a neuroma. Sometimes heel pain is nerve-related as well.

The probe generates a high-frequency, alternating current that causes heat necrosis of the nerve tissue. If successful, the end result for a neuroma is no pain, and it saves the patient from a more invasive surgery, which for neuromas often involves cutting out the portion of the nerve where the neuroma is located.

The treatment has shown up to an 80 percent success rate in eliminating pain from a Morton's neuroma and is also frequently used in the spine for back pain.

The Verdict: Excellent last-resort treatment to consider before open surgical techniques are used for neuroma pain and heel pain thought to be of nerve origin.

Cold Laser

Cold laser therapy, also known as low-level laser therapy (LLLT) is sometimes offered as a treatment for pain. It's a painless procedure using a wand-like applicator that emits a beam of light energy over the painful area. The energy is thought to be absorbed by the tissue to help reduce pain and inflammation. There are no studies to prove LLLT's effectiveness for a long duration but high-level studies show it can provide good short-term pain relief.

The Verdict: Cold laser is a good treatment when added to other treatments to help with short-term pain relief but not the best to be used as a solo treatment.

Smart Running Shoes

Altra began selling a "smart" running shoe during the spring 2016 season for $199. The Altra IQ is a pair of Bluetooth-equipped running shoes with sensors embedded in the soles to track all sorts of metrics specific to running. The shoe keeps tabs on standard stats such as your running distance, pace, time, and splits. But they also track your running cadence, how long your foot touches the ground on each stride, whether you favor one foot over the other, and which part of your foot hits the ground as you step.

A companion smartphone app analyzes the sensor data and provides feedback and suggestions along the way to help you become a better runner. It gives this feedback in real time, so you can make adjustments during your run.

The Verdict: I witnessed a demonstration of the Altra IQ at The Running Event in Austin, Texas, that touted it as the shoe to have. If the shoe proves to be successful with enough data that is applicable clinically, other shoe companies will probably follow suit. In the near future our running shoes may be able to give us feedback that can possibly help us stay healthy.

ElliptiGO

The ElliptiGO bike, created by Bryan Pate and Brent Teal, debuted in 2010. Bryan was unable to run due to injuries, and he didn't enjoy riding a regular bike or being inside on an elliptical trainer. The pair developed the combination of an elliptical machine and bike into the ElliptiGO.

There are four versions of the ElliptiGO. Some of the top runners in the world, including 2014 Boston Marathon champion and four-time Olympian Meb Keflezighi, regularly ride them. Keflezighi says replacing some of his running miles with time on the ElliptiGO has helped him stay injury-free and able to make the 2016 Olympic team at age forty.

The ElliptiGO is my favorite cross training tool. The bike challenges the core, provides a great aerobic workout, and is the closest exercise to running that allows you to be outside. Some bike shops and runner stores will offer a rental unit to try it out.

The Verdict: A great cross training alternative that's closer to the feeling of running than anything else. If, like me, you're a runner who isn't a fan of a traditional bicycle, you might enjoy the ElliptiGO.

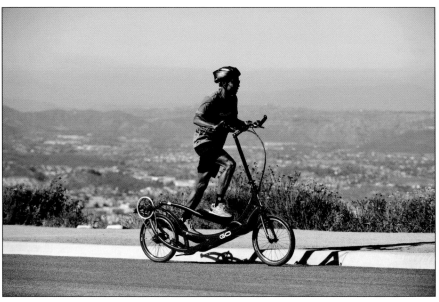

Meb Keflezighi training on an ElliptiGO.
Photo courtesy of ElliptiGO

Zero Runner

The Zero Runner is a home version of a new type of training tool. The device has some similarities to an elliptical machine but the user can more closely mimic the actual form of running. You can also move in reverse or more up and down. The movement and aerobic workout on the Zero Runner is similar to the ElliptiGO in that the "strides" are longer than on a standard elliptical machine. Another plus is that it's designed with a smaller footprint for home use.

The Verdict: Good choice for home use if running is limited due to the weather. It is more versatile than other machines.

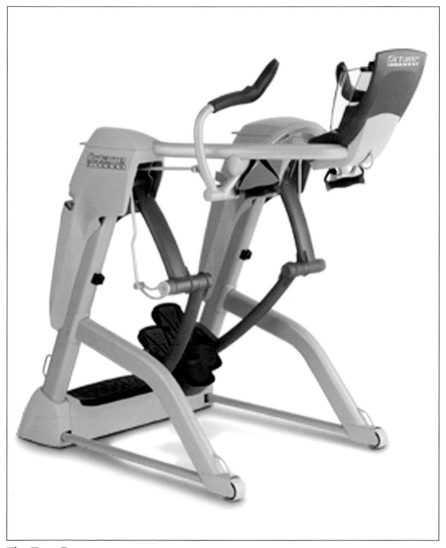

The Zero Runner.

Photo courtesy of Zero Runner

AlterG Treadmill

The AlterG is an anti-gravity treadmill that was designed to allow people with injuries or difficulty walking, such as after a stroke, to be able to exercise pain-free with less stress on the legs. The treadmill was designed using technology from NASA. The first prototype was tested by former champion marathoner, and now elite coach, Alberto Salazar in 2007.

The user wears a special pair of shorts that zips into an apron that surrounds your waist. This creates a chamber for the legs in which a differential air pressure technique developed by NASA allows the user to walk or run on the treadmill with as little as 20 percent of their body weight being transmitted to the legs. The AlterG allows people to run pain-free even in the presence of a broken bone or other injuries that would ordinarily not allow any weight-bearing activity.

With the least expensive model retailing for about $30,000, the cost of ownership is prohibitive for most people. But many hospitals and physician offices are buying the units, and runners can rent time on them to continue training. The AlterG website (www.AlterG.com) has a searchable list of units available for use. In my area the going rate is roughly a dollar per minute, with the price lower if you buy a package of uses.

The Verdict: I recommend the AlterG every day as an alternative to cross training for my injured runners. One of my patients sustained a stress fracture of her tibia eight weeks before the Chicago Marathon. She ran on the AlterG three times a week for six weeks along with swimming and biking, and was able to run and enjoy the marathon pain-free.

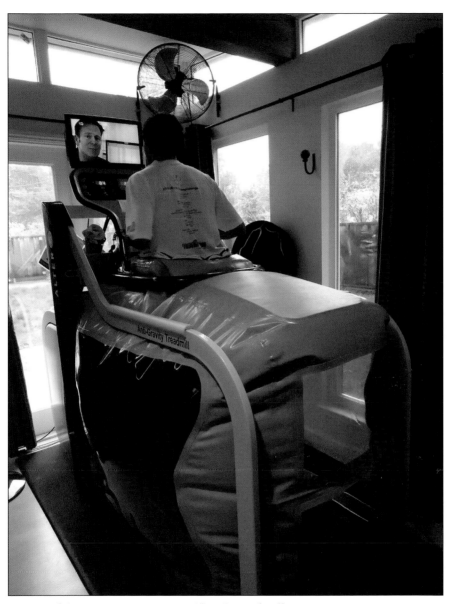

Dr. Amol Saxena training on an AlterG treadmill.

Photo courtesy of Dr. Amol Saxena

Correct Toes

Correct Toes were developed by Dr. Ray McClanahan, a Portland-based runner and podiatrist. They're slipped over the toes, and aim to progressively reverse deformities in the feet and the rest of the body by re-aligning a runner's toes and feet back into physiologically natural foot positions. This means that the widest part of the runner's feet will be at the ends of the toes, not at the balls of the feet.

Best results with Correct Toes are achieved when runners can run with their Correct Toes on. This requires that the runner fit their running footwear based upon the sock liner/insole measurement system.

The Verdict: An excellent tool to use to try to improve the strength and alignment of the foot, especially for those suffering chronic plantar fasciitis or other foot and ankle injuries.

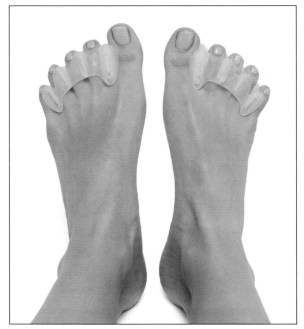

Photo courtesy of Dr. Ray McClanahan

3D Printed Orthotic Devices

Making foot orthotics with a 3D printer is already happening, but with some limitations and kinks that need to be worked out. Normally when an orthotic device is fabricated, the process—a plaster impression is made of the foot and sent to a lab where the device is fabricated—takes weeks to complete. 3D printers allow the foot to be scanned, and the specifications and modifications of the orthotic device to be inputted into the printer. The physician then feeds choice of material into the printer, and in a matter of hours the device is created by the printer.

The Verdict: A major current limitation is the ability of the scanner to capture all the same contours of the foot that plaster is able to do so well. This technology is definitely the future of custom foot orthotic fabrication. I anticipate the technology being readily available in your podiatrist's office within the next five to ten years.

Acknowledgments

First and foremost, I want to thank my parents, Bill and Donna Fullem. My two brothers, Mark and Kevin, and I played about ten different sports, and our parents almost never missed any of our events. In fact, of the more than 100 races I ran in high school, one or both of my parents were at every race but one. There are no better parents anywhere.

I've been fortunate to have learned from some great track coaches, starting at age ten with Sam Paniccia and Ralph Lupia. Rich Ambruso coached me in high school, and the late coach Art Gulden at Bucknell was one of the best distance coaches ever. I thank those two for helping to make me a better person. Thank you to Mike Barnow, my coach post-collegiately, not only for his coaching. Being on his Westchester Track Club enabled me to meet my wife and partner, Annemarie, on the track.

I want to thank Scott Douglas for asking me to write my first article for *Running Times* magazine in the early 1990s. We've shared many miles together, and I am grateful for the chance to work with him again on this book. Thank you to Weldon

Johnson for his contributions both as an injured athlete and for writing the foreword to this book. Weldon and his brother Robert are two of the best people in the track world.

There are many people who have helped to shape my professional life. I'm extremely grateful to two of my best friends, Dr. Rob Conenello and Dr. Amol Saxena, for their help with this book and with everything else in podiatry and life.

Words can't express how grateful I am to my wife, Annemarie Fullem. Her artwork makes this book better, and her physical therapy expertise has made me a better physician. Our two children, Aidan and Erin, are our greatest joy, and I'm so proud of them every day.

There are so many others who have helped me along the way. I'm hopeful this book can help runners run as much as they desire.

About the Author

Brian W. Fullem, DPM, is a nationally known sports podiatrist based in Clearwater, Florida. Dr. Fullem treats athletes of all abilities, from beginning runners up to Olympians, and has served as the team podiatrist for Yale University's track team and Sacred Heart University. He is a past board member of the American Academy of Podiatric Sports Medicine and is board-certified in foot surgery. Dr. Fullem ran a personal best of 14:25 for 5K on the track and was a member of the track and cross country teams at Bucknell University. He was a regular contributor for twenty years to the now-defunct *Running Times*. His articles on injury prevention and treatment were among the most read on the magazine's website.

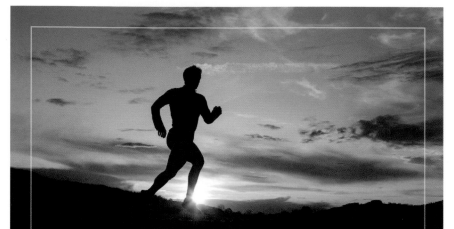

The
INNER
RUNNER

Running to a More Successful, Creative, and Confident You

JASON R. KARP, PhD

Jason R. Karp, PhD

The Inner Runner

Running to a More Successful, Creative, and Confident You

See how running provides a path to a better, more successful life.

Why are so many people drawn to running? Why is running the most common physical activity? What is it about running that empowers so many people? And how can runners harness that power to create a more meaningful life? *The Inner Runner* addresses these questions and a whole lot more. This book is not about how to get faster or run a marathon; rather, it explores how the simple act of putting one foot in front of the other helps you harness your creative powers. Learn about the psychological, emotional, cognitive, and spiritual benefits of running and introduce lifestyle changes based on the latest scientific research on running and its effects on hormones and the brain.

As a nationally recognized running and fitness coach with a PhD in exercise physiology, Jason Karp brings his expertise in science-based coaching to runners of all levels. He believes that running gives you a chance to discover, challenge, and bring out the best in yourself by impacting your creativity, focus, imagination, confidence, and health. Let *The Inner Runner* help you become not only a better runner but also a more creative, productive, and imaginative person.

Jason R. Karp, PhD, is one of America's foremost running experts, an established writer and author, an exercise physiologist, and creator of the Run-Fit Specialist certification. Dr. Karp has given dozens of international lectures and has been a featured speaker at most of the world's top fitness conferences and coaching clinics. His previous books include *Running a Marathon for Dummies, Running for Women, 101 Winning Racing Strategies for Runners,* and *101 Developmental Concepts & Workouts for Cross Country Runners.* He lives in San Diego, California.

$16.99 hardcover (Can. $23.99)
World (W) • CQ 30
ISBN 978-1-63450-795-0
5 ½" x 8 ¼" • 288 pages
Sports/Running
ebook ISBN 978-1-63450-801-8
APRIL

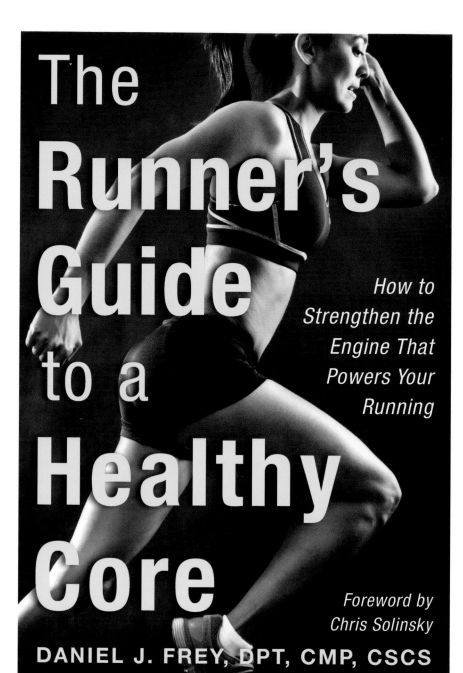

The Runner's Guide to a Healthy Core

How to Strengthen the Engine That Powers Your Running

Foreword by Chris Solinsky

DANIEL J. FREY, DPT, CMP, CSCS

Daniel J. Frey, DPT, CMS, CSCS

Foreword by Chris Solinsky

The Runner's Guide to a Healthy Core

How to Strengthen the Engine That Powers Your Running

The definitive guide for runners to attain and maintain peak core strength.

Every runner knows that you need more than just sturdy legs to achieve personal best performances and to stay injury free. To reach your optimal running potential, you need a strong and healthy core. Not only will having proper core strength give you toned abs and thighs, but it will also ensure that you maintain good form as your fatigue mounts, and ultimately it will decrease your chances of succumbing to devastating injury. In *The Runner's Guide to a Healthy Core*, celebrated orthopedic and champion runner Daniel Frey provides all the essential knowledge that is needed for achieving ideal core strength. Key pieces of information include:

- A detailed description of how the core functions when we run
- Illustrations of key core stretches and exercises
- A step-by-step guide to correct breathing while running
- Home remedies to ensure that soreness doesn't become injury
- And dozens more professionally endorsed tips and tactics!

Complete with dozens of color photographs and charts, *The Runner's Guide to a Healthy Core* contains all you'll ever need to gain and sustain a powerful and sturdy core strength.

Daniel J. Frey, DPT, CMP, CSCS, is a well-known orthopedic and sports physical therapist who specializes in the treatment of runners. Dan received his doctor of physical therapy degree from the University of New England. Prior to this, he attended the University of Delaware, where he completed his bachelor of science degree in exercise physiology. He lives in Portland, Maine.

Chris Solinsky is the former American record-holder in the ten thousand meters and a retired professional runner. He currently serves as head coach for the College of William & Mary's men's and women's track and cross country squads. He lives with his wife in Williamsburg, Virginia.

$16.99 paperback original (Can. $25.99)
World (W) • CQ 24
ISBN 978-1-5107-1138-9
6" x 9" • 176 pages
40 color photographs
Sports/Running
ebook ISBN 978-1-5107-1139-6
NOVEMBER

SLOW JOGGING

Lose Weight, Stay Healthy, and Have
Fun with Science-Based, Natural Running

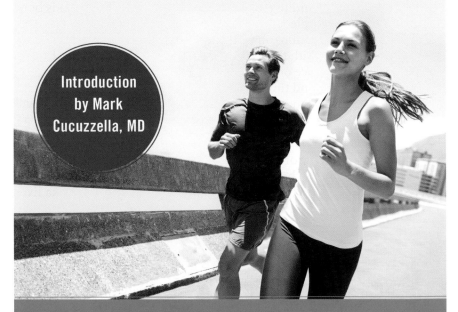

Introduction
by Mark
Cucuzzella, MD

HIROAKI TANAKA, PhD
WITH MAGDALENA JACKOWSKA

Hiroaki Tanaka, PhD, with Magdalena Jackowska

Introduction by Mark Cucuzzella, MD

Slow Jogging

Get Fit, Lose Weight, Stay Healthy, and Have Fun with Easy Running

The ultimate guide to enjoying injury-free running for life.

Running is America's most popular participatory sport, yet more than half of those who identify as runners get injured every year. Falling prey to injuries from overtraining, faulty form, poor eating, and improper footwear, many runners eventually, and reluctantly, abandon the sport for a less strenuous pastime. But for the first time in the United States, Hiroaki Tanaka's *Slow Jogging* demonstrates that there is an efficient, healthier, and pain-free approach to running for all ages and lifestyles.

Tanaka's method of easy running, or "slow jogging," is an injury-free approach to running that helps participants burn calories, lose weight, and even reverse the effects of type-2 diabetes. With easy-to-follow steps and colorful charts, *Slow Jogging* teaches runners to enjoy injury-free activity by:

- Maintaining a smiling, or niko niko in Japanese, pace that is both easy and enjoyable
- Landing on mid-foot, instead of on the heel
- Picking shoes with thin, flexible soles and no oversized heel
- Aiming for a pace of 180 steps per minute
- And trying to find time for activity every day
- Accessible to runners of all fitness levels and ages, *Slow Jogging* will inspire thousands more Americans to take up running.

Hiroaki Tanaka, PhD, is a professor at Fukuoka University, Japan, and the founder and director of the Fukuoka University Institute for Physical Activity. Currently he is the director of the Japanese Academic Running Society and an adviser to the Asashi running shoe company. Tanaka lives in Kyoto, Japan.

Magdalena Jackowska, a professional linguist, translator, and interpreter from Poland, is a research assistant at the Fukuoka University Institute for Physical Activity and a slow jogging instructor. She has completed more than twenty marathons and ultra-marathons all over the world—all in slow jogging style. Jackowska lives in Fukuoka, Japan.

$16.99 paperback original (Can. $23.99)
World (W) • CQ 30
ISBN 978-1-5107-0831-0
6" x 9" • 288 pages
Health/Fitness
ebook ISBN 978-1-5107-0832-7
APRIL